EVERYTHING ABOUT *ME*

A Guide for My Future Caregivers

Dee Marrella

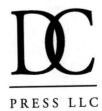

PRESS LLC

SANFORD • FLORIDA

For general information on our other products and services please contact our offices at 407-688-1156 and/or go to www.focusonethics.com or www.dcpress.com.

This book was set in Times New Roman and Arial
Cover Design and Composition by Debra Deysher

Everything About Me
ISBN: 978-1-932021-60-8

First DC Press Edition
Printed in the United States of America
10 9 8 7 6 5 4 3 2 1

This book is lovingly dedicated
to my mother, Beatrice Delia —
A happy person who suffered so much in her later years.

To my sisters,
Terry Nicoletti and Karen Wiesen —
Together, we tried our very best.

To my daughters,
Tammy Toso, Lani Martin and Robin Russo —
Your love and support during a very
trying time will never be forgotten.

To the love of my life, Len —
You encouraged me to care for my Mom.
You shared my stress and pain.
For this I am forever grateful.

To all who have shared your experiences with me.
You give me the inspiration to keep spreading
the message of loving care.

To future caregivers — May this book help make
the journey less stressful.

A NOTE TO MY CAREGIVERS

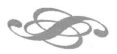

The information in this book is directed to those people — family, friends and strangers who might serve as my caregivers sometime in the future. When you read through the pages, keep in mind that I have made sincere efforts to help you understand me, but I've also attempted to understand you, my caregivers, and the important role you will play in my life in the future. Thanks in advance.

CONTENTS

v
— For My Caregivers —

xiii
— Why You Need To Complete This Book —

xv
— How to Complete this Book —

xix
— General Guidance for My Caregivers —

PART IV: FINANCES   91

"FAILING TO PLAN IS PLANNING TO FAIL"

~ Benjamin Franklin ~

WHY YOU NEED TO COMPLETE THIS BOOK

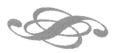

"This book is designed to be a true tool – one that you can count on in the event that you are one day in the hands of a caregiver. I have made every effort to include all aspects of your life.

Fill out only those sections that are meaningful and important to you now – those that will guarantee you have a voice in your own future well-being. You can update as needed later."

– Dee Marrella

HOW TO COMPLETE THIS BOOK

As you put down information about yourself, consider what you are doing as a "gift" for your loved ones. By recording aspects of your life and expressing your wishes and desires, you can reduce the fear of being a burden to others, while providing your future caregivers with less guilt and more peace of mind.

Planning for a major health crisis isn't typically on the top of anyone's "To Do List." Most of us can't fathom being incapacitated, unable to speak. But, in a split second, injury or illness can turn a perfectly healthy person into someone who is totally dependent. Your voice could be silenced. Others will speak for you. Question: Will that caregiver be a guardian angel with guidance and knowledge, or a confused interpreter, with little or no input from you?

The decision is yours. When you fill out this book, remember your future caregivers will be making decisions "with you, not for you."

> **NOTE:** Becoming a burden to one's family is a major anxiety for most long-term care patients.

If you are one of the fortunate Americans who can discuss your needs and directives with your future caregivers, this book can help open all kinds of doors. If possible, give a completed copy to the one(s) you hope will be your future caregiver(s). Ask them to become familiar with it. Invite questions. Suggest they take notes.

Remember: This is a living document – a work "in progress."

"SOMETIMES LIFE HAS A WAY OF PUTTING US ON OUR BACKS IN ORDER TO FORCE US TO LOOK UP."

~ Charles L. Allen ~

GENERAL GUIDANCE FOR MY CAREGIVERS

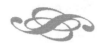

I pray that if I need care:

- I will be kept clean.

- I will be fed nutritious meals.

- I will be helped to keep my dignity as much as possible.

- I will obtain necessary medical care.

- I will not be treated as though I am already dead.

- I hope I will have the opportunity to continue to be around things I love – family, friends, jokes, music, movies, and good food until the day I do die!!

- I hope to be remembered for the love and support I tried to give to my family and friends. To be loved in return is to have true wealth.

While I am in a "rational" state, I do realize that if I am injured or ill:

- You cannot be with me 24 hours a day.

- You must go on with your life.

- You love me and will try to do your best to help keep me comfortable.

- At times, you will feel anger and guilt when I thrash out in frustration. I am not angry with you. I am angry and frustrated that I have become helpless and in need of assistance.

- You did not cause my illness or injury.

- You must also take care of the family and yourself.

Signed: _____

(Your signature here)

"WHERE WE LOVE IS HOME, HOME THAT OUR FEET MAY LEAVE, BUT NOT OUR HEARTS."

~ Oliver Wendell Holmes, Sr. ~

PART I

VITAL INFORMATION

The first section of this book contains essential information about ME that may be needed quickly, if I become ill suddenly or become a patient in a hospital or other healthcare facility.

Also included are relevant contacts and everything needed to insure that my family's home life can be maintained normally during my absence.

PERSONAL INFORMATION

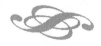

Last Name: _____

First Name: _____

Middle Name: _____

Maiden Name: (if applicable) _____

Nickname: _____

Named After: _____

Birth Date: _____

Place of Birth: _____

Location of BIRTH CERTIFICATE: _____

Current Address: _____

_____

_____

Current Telephone Number: _____

Cell Phone Number: _____

Email Address: _____

Marriage Location: _____

Date: _____

Location of MARRIAGE CERTIFICATE: _____

MILITARY HISTORY

(To be completed as needed to keep current)

I am serving/served from: _____ to: _____ in the:

_____	Army
_____	Air Force
_____	Navy
_____	Marines
_____	Coast Guard
_____	Other Service _____

My rank currently is / at discharge was:

_____

My most current rank date is/was (day, month, year)

_____

My discharge papers (DD214) are filed (location):

_____

I belong to the following veterans service organizations:

_____

_____

SPOUSE'S INFORMATION

Last Name: _____

First Name: _____

Middle Name: _____

Maiden Name: (if applicable) _____

Nickname: _____

Named After: _____

Birth Date: _____

Current Address: _____

_____

_____

Current Telephone Number: _____

Cell Phone Number: _____

Email Address: _____

Notes: _____

_____

_____

_____

VITAL INFORMATION

Previous Spouse (If Applicable):

Name:

Address:

Notes:

Parents Information:

Name:

Address:

Phone:

Notes:

CHILD'S PROFILE - Child #1

Name of Child : _____

Date of Birth: _____

Place of Birth: _____

Nickname: _____

Name of Doctor: _____

Name of Dentist: _____

Name of Optometrist: _____

List of Health Issues (Example: Allergies): _____

_____

_____

List of Medications: _____

_____

_____

Pharmacy Used: _____

Yearly Exams: _____

_____

_____

Location of Immunization Information: _____

VITAL INFORMATION

School Attended: _____

Address: _____

Phone #: _____

Principal's Name: _____

Legal Guardian(s): _____

Address: _____

Phone #: _____

Interests / Activities: _____

_____

_____

_____

_____

_____

Things He / She Fears: _____

_____

_____

Comforts Child Enjoys: _____

_____

_____

Additional Information / Issues: _____

_____

_____

CHILD'S PROFILE - Child #2

Name of Child : _____

Date of Birth: _____

Place of Birth: _____

Nickname: _____

Name of Doctor: _____

Name of Dentist: _____

Name of Optometrist: _____

List of Health Issues (Example: Allergies) _____

_____

_____

List of Medications: _____

_____

_____

Pharmacy Used: _____

Yearly Exams: _____

_____

_____

Location of Immunization Information: _____

VITAL INFORMATION

School Attended: _____

Address: _____

Phone #: _____

Principal's Name: _____

Legal Guardian(s): _____

Address: _____

Phone #: _____

Interests / Activities: _____

_____

_____

_____

_____

_____

Things He / She Fears: _____

_____

_____

Comforts Child Enjoys: _____

_____

_____

Additional Information / Issues: _____

_____

_____

CHILD'S PROFILE - Child #3

Name of Child : _____

Date of Birth: _____

Place of Birth: _____

Nickname: _____

Name of Doctor: _____

Name of Dentist: _____

Name of Optometrist: _____

List of Health Issues (Example: Allergies) _____

_____

_____

List of Medications: _____

_____

_____

Pharmacy Used: _____

Yearly Exams: _____

_____

_____

Location of Immunization Information: _____

VITAL INFORMATION

School Attended: _____

Address: _____

Phone #: _____

Principal's Name: _____

Legal Guardian(s): _____

Address: _____

Phone #: _____

Interests / Activities: _____

_____

_____

_____

_____

_____

Things He / She Fears: _____

_____

_____

Comforts Child Enjoys: _____

_____

_____

Additional Information / Issues: _____

_____

_____

IMPORTANT HOUSEHOLD INFORMATION & CONTACTS

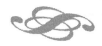

Newspaper Delivery Contacts: _____

Garbage Collection Days: _____

Trash/Recycling Collection Days:_____

Location of Circuit Breaker or Fusebox: _____

_____

Alarm System:

    Contact: _____

    Address: _____

    Phone #: _____

    Location of:

    Arming Code: _____

    Disarming Code:_____

Location of Water Shut-offs: _____

_____

EVERYTHING ABOUT *ME*

—— ✧ ——

IMPORTANT KEYS:

Keys to House/Apartment:

Location/Comments: _____

_____

Keys to Car(s):

Location/Comments: _____

_____

_____

Keys to Safety Deposit Box:

Location/Comments: _____

_____

Keys to Office:

Location/Comments: _____

_____

Storage Company:

Location/Comments: _____

_____

Other Important Keys:

Location/Comments: _____

_____

VITAL INFORMATION

Electric Company:

    Name: _____

    Phone: _____

Gas Company:

    Name: _____

    Phone: _____

Phone / Internet / Cable:

    Name: _____

    Phone: _____

Water Company:

    Name: _____

    Phone: _____

Plumber:

    Name: _____

    Phone: _____

Electrician:

    Name: _____

    Phone: _____

Lawn Maintenance Person:

    Name: _____

    Phone: _____

Pool Maintenance Person:

    Name: _____

    Phone: _____

Snow Removal:

    Name: _____

    Phone: _____

Heating and Air Conditioning Company:

    Name: _____

    Phone: _____

Pest Control:

    Name: _____

    Phone: _____

Computer Repair:

    Name: _____

    Phone: _____

Auto Repair:

    Name: _____

    Phone: _____

Location and information for proper use of fire extinguishers:

_____

_____

_____

Turn-off locations for:

    Electricity: _____

    Gas: _____

    Furnace: _____

CAR MAINTENANCE

1. Location of vehicle registration:

    _____

2. Location of auto insurance policy:

    _____

3. State inspection due date :

    _____

4. Location of extra set of car keys:

    _____

5. Tire pressure:

    _____

6. Gasoline type:

    _____

7. Oil Brand: _____ Weight: _____

8. Maintenance service station/dealership:

    Service consultant: _____

    Phone Number: _____

    Address: _____

    Warranty Programs: _____

9. Car Payments: (Monthly)

    Company: _____ Amount: _____

CARING FOR MY PETS IN A TIME OF EMERGENCY

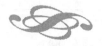

PET #1

Type of pet: _____

Name of pet: _____

Pet named _____, does NOT like the following
(thought it important to let you know): _____

_____

Specific Health Issues: _____

_____

_____

Medications: _____

_____

Location of Vaccination Information: _____

_____

Suggestion: Consider placing your cell phone number on your pet's collar or consider having a microchip implanted.

VITAL INFORMATION

Veterinarian: Name: _____

Phone: _____

Address: _____

_____

Pet Groomer: Name: _____

Phone: _____

Address: _____

_____

Kennel: Name: _____

Phone: _____

Address: _____

_____

Name / phone number of individual who could care for pet temporarily:

Name: _____

Phone: _____

Address: _____

_____

Brand of General Pet Food:

Dry: _____

_____

Wet: _____

_____

Brand of Biscuits: _____

Brand of Special Treats: _____

Exercise habits: _____

_____

_____

Where he/she prefers to sleep: _____

_____

_____

Would you like your pet to visit you if possible?

_____ Yes   _____ No

Arrangements for permanent care for my pet – to assure that my pet is loved and properly cared for:

_____

_____

_____

_____

_____

_____

_____

_____

_____

_____

_____

_____

CARING FOR MY PETS IN
A TIME OF EMERGENCY

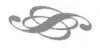

PET #2

Type of pet: _____

Name of pet: _____

Pet named _____, does NOT like the following
(thought it important to let you know): _____

_____

Specific Health Issues: _____

_____

_____

Medications: _____

_____

Location of Vaccination Information: _____

_____

Suggestion: Affordable health insurance for pets is becoming acceptable among serious pet owners. You can get a list of providers from your local pet shop or by searching the Internet.

Veterinarian: Name: _____

Phone: _____

Address: _____

_____

Pet Groomer: Name: _____

Phone: _____

Address: _____

_____

Kennel: Name: _____

Phone: _____

Address: _____

_____

Name / phone number of individual who could care for pet temporarily:

Name: _____

Phone: _____

Address: _____

_____

Brand of General Pet Food:

Dry: _____

_____

Wet: _____

_____

Brand of Biscuits: _____

Brand of Special Treats: _____

VITAL INFORMATION

Exercise habits: _____

_____

_____

Where he/she prefers to sleep: _____

_____

_____

Would you like your pet to visit you if possible?

_____ Yes   _____ No

Arrangements for permanent care for my pet – to assure that my pet is loved and properly cared for:

_____

_____

_____

_____

_____

_____

_____

_____

_____

_____

_____

_____

CARING FOR MY PETS IN
A TIME OF EMERGENCY

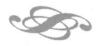

PET #3

Type of pet: _____

Name of pet: _____

Pet named _____, does NOT like the following
(thought it important to let you know): _____

_____

Specific Health Issues: _____

_____

_____

Medications: _____

_____

Location of Vaccination Information: _____

_____

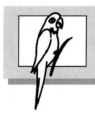

Suggestion: Any papers/proof that pets have current vaccinations should be kept in a folder/large envelope and clearly marked.

24

VITAL INFORMATION

Veterinarian: Name: _____

                    Phone: _____

                    Address: _____

_____

Pet Groomer: Name: _____

                    Phone: _____

                    Address: _____

_____

Kennel: Name: _____

                    Phone: _____

                    Address: _____

_____

Name / phone number of individual who could care for pet temporarily:

                    Name: _____

                    Phone: _____

                    Address: _____

_____

Brand of General Pet Food:

                    Dry: _____

_____

                    Wet: _____

_____

Brand of Biscuits: _____

Brand of Special Treats: _____

Exercise habits:

_____

_____

_____

Where he/she prefers to sleep:

_____

_____

_____

Would you like your pet to visit you if possible?

_____ Yes   _____ No

Arrangements for permanent care for my pet – to assure that my pet is loved and properly cared for:

_____

_____

_____

_____

_____

_____

_____

_____

_____

_____

_____

"BEFORE A CATASTROPHE, WE CAN'T IMAGINE COPING WITH THE BURDENS THAT MIGHT CONFRONT US IN A DIRE MOMENT. THEN WHEN THAT MOMENT ARRIVES, WE SUDDENLY FIND THAT WE HAVE RESOURCES INSIDE US THAT WE KNEW NOTHING ABOUT."

~ Christopher Reeve ~

PART II

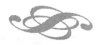

ABOUT ME

This section contains important information about me, including personal statistics, medical history and my preferences for everyday living. If you understand my health and medical status, you know one aspect of who I am. Additionally, I have many things that I like, some that I dislike and some things that I want nothing to do with. There are tastes, smells, sounds and images, colors, books, movies, games and so many other things that really describe who I am. When you read the following, please know that I have given lots of thought to what is written here. I believe these bits of information about me will help you understand the real me.

PRIORITIES FOR CARE

Address each section as completely as possible. Use pencil for any information that may change.

> ***Note:** Update this section whenever there is a change in medications, attending physicians, etc. Make certain your entries in this section and your legal documents (Living Will, Health Care Directive) are consistent.

Making medical decisions for a loved one can be an anguishing task for a caretaker.

MY PROFILE

Listed below are my personal statistics and profile:

Statistics:

Height: _____

Weight: _____

Birthdate: (DD/MM/YYYY) _____

Eye Color: _____

Hair Color: _____

Shoe Size: _____

Current Date: _____

Health issues of concern to me: Examples: Asthma, Tinnitus, IBS

_____

_____

_____

My favorite civilian healthcare providers: _____

_____

*Note: Provide specific contact information about civilian providers later in this section.

PERSONAL MEDICAL HISTORY

The following is a list of known medical conditions/major injuries that should be noted:

Name of illness/injury:

Age of occurrence: _____

Type of treatment: _____

_____

_____

Long-term impact: _____

_____

_____

Name of illness/injury:

Age of occurrence: _____

Type of treatment: _____

_____

_____

Long-term impact: _____

_____

_____

ABOUT ME

Name of illness/injury:

Age of occurrence: _____

Type of treatment: _____

_____

_____

Long-term impact: _____

_____

_____

Name of illness/injury:

Age of occurrence: _____

Type of treatment: _____

_____

_____

Long-term impact: _____

_____

_____

Name of illness/injury:

Age of occurrence: _____

Type of treatment: _____

_____

_____

Long-term impact: _____

_____

_____

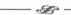

Physical problems I have and medications I take for them (include all prescription and over-the-counter drugs):

Condition: _____

Name of Drug(s): _____

Dosage: _____

# of Doses / Daily: _____

Condition: _____

Name of Drug(s): _____

Dosage: _____

# of Doses / Daily: _____

Drug & medical allergies: (example: Latex, iodine, tape)

_____

_____

_____

Environmental allergies and medications taken (include all prescription and over-the-counter drugs):

Allergy: _____

Name of Drug: _____

Dosage: _____

# of Doses / Daily: _____

Allergy: _____

Name of Drug: _____

Dosage: _____

# of Doses / Daily: _____

IF I HAD A TERMINAL ILLNESS

_____ I would want to know.

_____ I would not want to know.

Comments on above:

_____

_____

_____

_____

_____

_____

_____

_____

_____

_____

_____

_____

_____

_____

Would I want you to request any hospital or doctor to keep me alive through extreme means if I were suffering?

_____ Yes   _____ No

- Is it legally documented somewhere?

    Yes   _____
    No   _____
    Location   _____

- I do have a Living Will

    Yes   _____
    No   _____
    Location   _____

- I do have a Healthcare Directive

    Yes   _____
    No   _____
    Location   _____

ABOUT ME

I want the following to be done:

If my heart stops, I do____ do not____ want CPR (cardiopulmonary resuscitation).

I do____ do not____ want to be placed on any mechanical breathing apparatus.

I do____ do not____ want to have any blood transfusions.

I do____ do not____ want any intravenous food administered.

I do____ do not____ want any liquids administered intravenously.

If I am transported to a healthcare facility and placed on life support, I do____ do not ____ want it stopped at the directive of my representative(s).

Comments on this subject:

If I am unable to communicate, I want my wishes followed regardless if you agree:

Yes   _____

No   _____

Explain   _____

_____
Spouse's Signature

I Would Like To Be An Organ Donor:

_____ Yes   _____ No

Comments on Organ Donation:

_____

_____

_____

_____

_____

_____

_____

Any Special Requests Regarding Organ Donation:

_____

_____

_____

_____

_____

Where Official Documentation is Located:

_____

_____

_____

MY FAVORITE HEALTHCARE PROVIDERS INCLUDE

Physician: Name: _____

Phone: _____

Address: _____

_____

Dentist: Name: _____

Phone: _____

Address: _____

_____

Podiatrist: Name: _____

Phone: _____

Address: _____

_____

Optometrist: Name: _____

Phone: _____

Address: _____

_____

Optician: Name: _____

              Phone: _____

              Address: _____

                        _____

Pharmacy: Name: _____

              Phone: _____

              Address: _____

                        _____

Hospital: Name: _____

              Phone: _____

              Address: _____

                        _____

Insurance   Name: _____

Agent 1:   Phone: _____

              Address: _____

                        _____

Insurance   Name: _____

Agent 2:   Phone: _____

              Address: _____

                        _____

Other: Name: _____

              Phone: _____

              Address: _____

                        _____

DOCTORS, HOSPITALS, OTHER PROFESSIONALS THAT I <u>NEVER</u> WANT TO GO BACK TO

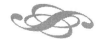

Name: _____

Phone: _____

Address: _____

Reasons _____

_____

Name: _____

Phone: _____

Address: _____

Reasons _____

_____

Name: _____

Phone: _____

Address: _____

Reasons _____

_____

FAMILY INVOLVEMENT

What options do I prefer for my care? (For instance, having loved ones or care professionals assist me at home or moving to an assisted living facility?)

_____

_____

_____

_____

_____

_____

_____

_____

_____

_____

_____

_____

_____

*Note: Only 8% of Americans have talked about these issues with spouses or partners.

How will I pay for my care if necessary?

_____

_____

_____

_____

_____

_____

_____

_____

_____

_____

_____

_____

_____

_____

_____

_____

_____

_____

_____

_____

_____

_____

_____

_____

_____

MY TYPICAL DAY

I think it is important for any caregiver to understand what my typical day is like, and how much it means that these routine activities and rituals be maintained as much as possible.

- I am a____day person____night person (Check proper response.)

- I usually wake at_____AM.

- I like eating breakfast at_____AM.

- Most mornings I enjoy: (examples: working on car, watching TV, video games)

  _____

  _____

  _____

- I like to eat my lunch at_____AM or PM.

- I enjoy an afternoon nap at_____PM.

- Most afternoons I enjoy:

  _____

  _____

  _____

ABOUT ME

- I like eating dinner at_____PM.

- After dinner I enjoy:

  _____

  _____

  _____

  _____

  _____

- I usually get ready for bed at_____PM.

- I like to:

  Read in bed_____
  Watch TV in bed_____
  Go right to sleep_____

- I communicate daily with the following people:

Name: _____

Relationship: _____

Phone # _____

E-mail address: _____

Name: _____

Relationship: _____

Phone # _____

E-mail address: _____

EVERYTHING ABOUT *ME*

Name: _____

Relationship: _____

Phone # _____

E-mail address: _____

Name: _____

Relationship: _____

Phone # _____

E-mail address: _____

Name: _____

Relationship: _____

Phone # _____

E-mail address: _____

Name: _____

Relationship: _____

Phone # _____

E-mail address: _____

Name: _____

Relationship: _____

Phone # _____

E-mail address: _____

MY FAVORITE FOODS

For Breakfast:

_____

_____

_____

_____

_____

For Lunch:

_____

_____

_____

_____

_____

For Dinner:

_____

_____

_____

_____

_____

FOOD CHOICES

Foods I love and would eat at any time:

_____

_____

_____

_____

_____

Foods I absolutely hate and would never eat:

_____

_____

_____

_____

_____

Foods I am allergic to:

_____

_____

_____

_____

_____

My favorite snack foods include:

_____

_____

_____

_____

_____

ABOUT ME

My favorites:

Candy: _____

_____

Cake: _____

_____

Pie: _____

_____

Ice Cream: _____

_____

Fast Foods: _____

_____

Soups: _____

_____

Salads/Salad
Dressings: _____

_____

Entrees: _____

_____

_____

_____

_____

My thoughts on organic foods:

_____

_____

_____

_____

_____

Ethnic foods I do/do not enjoy:

_____

_____

_____

_____

_____

_____

_____

Favorite Beverages:

Non-Alcoholic:
_____

_____

_____

_____

Alcoholic:
_____

_____

_____

_____

HOBBIES AND PERSONAL INTERESTS

My five top hobbies:

1. _____
2. _____
3. _____
4. _____
5. _____

My talents include:

Musical Instruments I play (or played):

_____
_____
_____
_____
_____

Singing Ability:

_____
_____
_____
_____
_____

Acting Ability:

_____

_____

_____

_____

_____

Other Interests / Talents / Skills:

_____

_____

_____

_____

_____

_____

_____

_____

_____

_____

_____

_____

_____

_____

_____

_____

_____

_____

ENTERTAINMENT PREFERENCES

Types of TV shows I enjoy:

_____

_____

_____

_____

Favorite movies and videos I enjoy viewing:

_____

_____

_____

_____

Favorite TV networks:

_____

_____

_____

_____

Sports I like to watch (on TV or in person):

Sport   Favorite Team

_____   _____

_____   _____

_____   _____

_____   _____

Favorite Sports Figures:

_____

_____

_____

_____

_____

Favorite TV stars:

_____

_____

_____

_____

_____

Favorite Movie Stars:

_____

_____

_____

_____

_____

ABOUT ME

Types of TV shows / Movies I do not enjoy:

_____

_____

_____

_____

Radio programs I enjoy:

_____

_____

_____

_____

Radio programs I do not enjoy:

_____

_____

_____

_____

Music I enjoy listening to:

_____

_____

_____

_____

Music that gives me a headache:

_____

_____

_____

_____

Favorite singers:

_____

_____

_____

_____

Newspapers and magazines I enjoy reading:

_____

_____

_____

_____

My favorite authors:

_____

_____

_____

_____

ABOUT ME

Video games I enjoy:

_____

_____

_____

_____

_____

_____

_____

Card games I enjoy:

_____

_____

_____

Board games I enjoy:

_____

_____

_____

Other games:

_____

_____

IF PLANNING A DAY OR EVENING OUT, THIS IS WHAT I WOULD LIKE TO DO

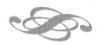

In town:

_____

_____

_____

_____

_____

_____

Out of town:

_____

_____

_____

_____

_____

_____

FAVORITE PRODUCT BRANDS

Toothpaste: _____

Mouthwash: _____

Deodorant: _____

Soap: _____

Shampoo / Conditioner: _____

Cologne: _____

Shaving Products / Razor: _____

I prefer to take: (Check one)

    Shower: _____

    Bath: _____

Products I am allergic to:

    1. _____

    2. _____

    3. _____

Female:

    Perfume: _____

    Deodorant: _____

    Brand(s) of Makeup Preferred: _____

    _____

    Hairspray: _____

Bedtime clothing I am most comfortable wearing:

Pajamas   _____

Underwear   _____

Warm-ups   _____

Other   _____

My favorite bed pillow (Check One):

Soft   _____

Medium   _____

Hard   _____

Other   _____

Clothes I am most comfortable in:

_____

_____

_____

Fabrics that irritate my skin:

1. _____

2. _____

3. _____

4. None

Other Personal Care Directions:

_____

_____

_____

_____

RELIGIOUS AFFILIATION

Church, Synagogue, Mosque, Temple, Other Religious Facility:

_____

Address: _____

Telephone #: _____

E-mail address: _____

Web site: _____

Key Contact Person(s):

     Name: _____

     Cell Phone: _____

     Name: _____

     Cell Phone: _____

Describe Attendance (include time of day, seating area and other important points):

_____

_____

_____

_____

_____

_____

_____

_____

Describe Participation (such as choir, usher, teacher, etc.):

_____

_____

_____

_____

_____

_____

_____

My favorite religious passages, scriptures, meditations, readings:

_____

_____

_____

The importance of religion in my life:

_____

_____

_____

_____

_____

_____

_____

_____

_____

_____

_____

"YOU DON'T GET TO CHOOSE HOW YOU'RE GOING TO DIE, OR WHEN. YOU CAN ONLY DECIDE HOW YOU'RE GOING TO LIVE NOW!"

~ Joan Baez ~

PART I I I

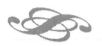

REFLECTIONS

Messages
For My
Loved Ones
&
Personal Thoughts,
Remembrances and Reflections

Advice or philosophy of life I want to pass on to my children and/or grandchildren:

_____

_____

_____

_____

_____

_____

_____

_____

_____

_____

_____

_____

_____

_____

_____

_____

_____

_____

_____

_____

Advice or philosophy - continued:

How I would like to be remembered:

_____

_____

_____

_____

_____

_____

_____

_____

_____

_____

_____

_____

_____

_____

_____

_____

_____

_____

REGRETS IN MY LIFE

If I had to do it all over again . . .

Regrets I have:

_____

_____

_____

_____

_____

_____

_____

_____

_____

_____

_____

_____

_____

_____

_____

_____

_____

_____

_____

_____

Special interests I wish I had pursued:

_____

_____

_____

_____

_____

_____

What is really important in life:

_____

_____

_____

_____

_____

_____

_____

_____

_____

_____

CHILDREN

#1. Full name   _____

Date of Birth   _____

Birthplace   _____

A fond memory or two spent together:

_____

_____

_____

_____

A message for: _____ (child's name)

CHILDREN

#2.   Full name _____

Date of Birth _____

Birthplace _____

A fond memory or two spent together:

_____

_____

_____

_____

A message for: _____ (child's name)

CHILDREN

#3.   Full name

       Date of Birth

       Birthplace

A fond memory or two spent together:

A message for: _____ (child's name)

A Letter For My Loved Ones

*PARENTS' INFORMATION

MATERNAL:

Mother:
   Name: _____
   Current Address: _____

_____

   Current Phone #: _____ Cell: _____
   Email/Web Site: _____

Father:
   Name: _____
   Current Address: _____

_____

   Current Phone #: _____ Cell: _____
   Email/Web Site: _____

PATERNAL:

Mother:
   Name: _____
   Current Address: _____

_____

   Current Phone #: _____ Cell: _____
   Email/Web Site: _____

Father:
   Name: _____
   Current Address: _____

_____

   Current Phone #: _____ Cell: _____
   Email/Web Site: _____

*If living

My Chart of Descendants

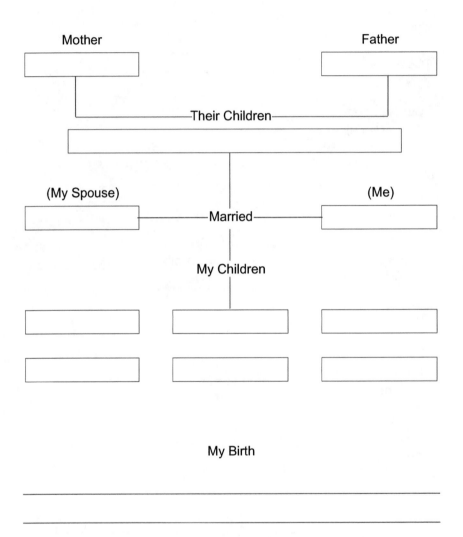

Mother

Father

Their Children

(My Spouse)

(Me)

Married

My Children

My Birth

"ONE PERSON CARING ABOUT ANOTHER REPRESENTS LIFE'S GREATEST VALUE."

~ *John Rohn* ~

EDUCATION

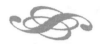

Elementary School

Name: _____

Address: _____

_____

_____

Junior High or Middle School

Name: _____

Address: _____

_____

_____

High School

Name: _____

Address: _____

_____

_____

REFLECTIONS

College / University

Undergraduate:

Location: _____

Major: _____

Minor: _____

Honors: _____

Graduate:

Location: _____

Major: _____

Degree Received: _____

Trade School:

Location: _____

Major: _____

Additional Educational Information:

_____

_____

_____

_____

_____

JOBS OR CAREER HISTORY

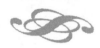

Company Name:

    Location: _____

    Job Title/Description: _____

    Years Employed: _____

Company Name:

    Location: _____

    Job Title/Description: _____

    Years Employed: _____

Company Name:

    Location: _____

    Job Title/Description: _____

    Years Employed: _____

Comments: _____

_____

_____

_____

_____

"ALWAYS REMEMBER THAT YOU ARE ABSOLUTELY UNIQUE – JUST LIKE EVERYONE ELSE."

~ Margaret Mead ~

FAMILY HOLIDAYS/ TRADITIONS

NOTE: For many people, Thanksgiving and Halloween are typical holidays that are observed. However, since there are many holidays throughout any given year, and considering that we all celebrate different ones in our own family structure, (e.g., Christmas, Easter, Hanukkah, Ramadan, Kwanzaa) please fill in the ones you honor.

REFLECTIONS

My favorite holiday:

_____

_____

_____

_____

_____

_____

_____

Why this holidays has always been so special:

_____

_____

_____

_____

_____

_____

_____

_____

_____

_____

_____

_____

Holiday

Family Tradition Observed _____

_____

_____

_____

_____

_____

_____

Holiday

Family Tradition Observed _____

_____

_____

_____

_____

_____

_____

Holiday

Family Tradition Observed _____

_____

_____

_____

_____

_____

_____

REFLECTIONS

What I love to do on my favorite holiday:

_____

_____

_____

_____

_____

_____

_____

Holiday vacation(s) I have enjoyed the most (such as a visit to the seashore, to the mountains, taking a cruise, etc.):

_____

_____

_____

_____

_____

_____

_____

_____

_____

_____

_____

FAMILY MEMORIES

What I know of my family's history prior to my birth:

_____

_____

_____

_____

_____

_____

_____

_____

_____

_____

_____

_____

_____

_____

_____

_____

_____

_____

REFLECTIONS

Who most influenced my life (How?):

_____

_____

_____

_____

_____

_____

_____

_____

_____

_____

_____

_____

_____

_____

_____

_____

_____

_____

_____

_____

The one thing I did in my life that made me the happiest or most proud – my greatest accomplishment:

_____

_____

_____

_____

_____

_____

_____

_____

_____

_____

_____

_____

_____

_____

_____

_____

_____

_____

_____

_____

_____

_____

"ADVANCE PLANNING IS LIKE TAKING A DEEP BREATH BEFORE THE PLUNGE. IT'S THE CALM BEFORE THE STORM. AND THAT'S WHEN IT'S TIME TO PREPARE, WHILE ITS CALM TO INSURE SUCCESS NO MATTER WHAT UNEXPECTED STORMS MIGHT COME.

~ Robin Crow ~

PART I V

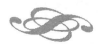

MY FINANCES

My financial information is obviously important and highly personal. What I provide on the following pages is intended to aid and assist those who are caring for me. I appreciate that this information is respected and used only for the purpose of making my life and my caregivers' lives easier.

IMPORTANT HOUSEHOLD INFORMATION & CONTACTS

Important Names and Phone Numbers (this list includes individuals you deal with).

Bank:

Name: _____

Phone: _____

Address: _____

_____

List all account names: _____

_____

_____

_____

_____

_____

Financial Planner:

Name: _____

Phone: _____

Address: _____

_____

FINANCES

Attorney:

Name: _____

Phone: _____

Address: _____

_____

Accountant:

Name: _____

Phone: _____

Address: _____

_____

Tax Preparer:

Name: _____

Phone: _____

Address: _____

_____

Location of Previous Tax Records:

Name: _____

Phone: _____

Address: _____

_____

*Note: Tax records should be retained for 7 years.

Broker:

Name: _____

Phone: _____

Address: _____

_____

Money Market Fund:

Name: _____

Phone: _____

Address: _____

Account Names / Bank Name: _____

_____

Name: _____

Phone: _____

Address: _____

Account Names / Bank Name: _____

_____

Name: _____

Phone: _____

Address: _____

Account Names / Bank Name: _____

_____

FINANCES

401K / Thrift Savings Plan:

Name: _____

Phone: _____

Address: _____

_____

IRA's

Name: _____

Phone: _____

Address: _____

Account Names: _____

_____

Name: _____

Phone: _____

Address: _____

Account Names: _____

_____

Funeral Home:

Name: _____

Phone: _____

Address: _____

_____

Safety Deposit Box:

Name: _____

Phone: _____

Address: _____

_____

Box #: _____

_____

Pension or Retirement Plans (List Details):

Military:

_____

_____

_____

_____

_____

_____

Retirement:

_____

_____

_____

_____

_____

_____

PERSONAL & BUSINESS AFFAIRS

Locating and understanding where important papers can be found (provide location, contact person if needed, contact phone numbers):

Original Will:

Location: _____

Executor(s)

Name: _____
Phone: _____
Address: _____

Name: _____
Phone: _____
Address: _____

Power of Attorney (If different than above):

Name: _____
Phone: _____
Address: _____

Name: _____
Phone: _____
Address: _____

Copies of Wills

Name: _____

Phone: _____

Address: _____

Name: _____

Phone: _____

Address: _____

Trusts:

Location: _____

Type: _____

Name: _____

Phone: _____

Address: _____

Checking Account(s):

Name: _____

Phone: _____

Address: _____

Account Name/Bank: _____

Savings Account(s):

Name: _____

Phone: _____

Address: _____

Account Name/Bank: _____

FINANCES

Real Estate (Deeds, Mortgages, Rental Agreements)

Name/Location: _____

Phone: _____

Address: _____

_____

Contact: _____

_____

Titles (Automobile and Other Vehicles)

Name/Location: _____

Phone: _____

Address: _____

_____

Contact: _____

_____

Name/Location: _____

Phone: _____

Address: _____

_____

Contact: _____

_____

Stock Certificates:

Name: _____

Phone: _____

Address: _____

Owners Name: _____

Name: _____

Phone: _____

Address: _____

Owners Name: _____

Name: _____

Phone: _____

Address: _____

Owners Name: _____

Name: _____

Phone: _____

Address: _____

Owners Name: _____

FINANCES

Bonds:

Name: _____

Phone: _____

Address: _____

Owners Name: _____

Name: _____

Phone: _____

Address: _____

Owners Name: _____

Name: _____

Phone: _____

Address: _____

Owners Name: _____

Name: _____

Phone: _____

Address: _____

Owners Name: _____

MILITARY BENEFITS

Active Duty Benefits: (List)

Name of Insured: _____

_____

_____

_____

_____

_____

Active Duty: See your base, post or command headquarters for further information about your benefits.

Retirees: Contact the Veterans Administration by phone at 1-800-827-1000, for hearing impaired, use Telecommunications Device for the Deaf (TDD): 1-800-829-4833, or visit their web site at http://www.va.gov. You can get Free Military Handbooks on these subjects at: http://www.militaryhandbooks.com.

Retiree Benefits: (List)

Name of Insured: _____

_____

_____

_____

_____

_____

INSURANCE POLICIES

Life Insurance:

Name of Insurance Company _____

Insurance Company Phone # _____

Policy # _____

Group # _____

Member ID # (If Applicable) _____

Co-pays # (If Applicable) _____

Address of Company _____

_____

Location of Policy _____

Name of Insurance Company _____

Insurance Company Phone # _____

Policy # _____

Group # _____

Member ID # (If Applicable) _____

Co-pays # (If Applicable) _____

Address of Company _____

_____

Location of Policy _____

House/Real Estate/Rental Property Insurance:

Name of Insurance Company _____

Insurance Company Phone # _____

Policy # _____

Group # _____

Member ID # (If Applicable) _____

Co-pays # (If Applicable) _____

Address of Company _____

Location of Policy _____

Automotive Insurance:

Name of Insurance Company _____

Insurance Company Phone # _____

Policy # _____

Group # _____

Member ID # (If Applicable) _____

Co-pays # (If Applicable) _____

Address of Company _____

Location of Policy _____

Health Insurance:

Name of Insurance Company _____

Insurance Company Phone # _____

Policy # _____

Group # _____

Member ID # (If Applicable) _____

Co-pays # (If Applicable) _____

Address of Company _____

Location of Policy _____

FINANCES

Dental Insurance:

Name of Insurance Company _____

Insurance Company Phone # _____

Policy # _____

Group # _____

Member ID # (If Applicable) _____

Co-pays # (If Applicable) _____

Address of Company _____

Location of Policy _____

Vision Insurance:

Name of Insurance Company _____

Insurance Company Phone # _____

Policy # _____

Group # _____

Member ID # (If Applicable) _____

Co-pays # (If Applicable) _____

Address of Company _____

Location of Policy _____

Other Insurance: (i.e. Personal Property, Umbrella Policy, etc.)

Name of Insurance Company _____

Insurance Company Phone # _____

Policy # _____

Group # _____

Member ID # (If Applicable) _____

Co-pays # (If Applicable) _____

Address of Company _____

Location of Policy _____

Long-Term Health Insurance:

Name of Insurance Company _____

Insurance Company Phone # _____

Policy # _____

Group # _____

Member ID # (If Applicable) _____

Co-pays # (If Applicable) _____

Address of Company _____

Location of Policy _____

Cash or Long-Term Care Policy that covers costs:

Name of Insurance Company _____

Insurance Company Phone # _____

Policy # _____

Group # _____

Member ID # (If Applicable) _____

Co-pays # (If Applicable) _____

Address of Company _____

Location of Policy _____

Dedicated Cash Account:

Location: _____

Contact _____

Phone _____

Address _____

_____

Comments _____

_____

LIST OF ASSETS

Home:

Address: _____

Purchase price: _____

Current value: _____

Last Appraisal Date: _____

Location of Deed(s) _____

Automobile(s):

Make/Model: _____

Year: _____

Location of Title: _____

Make/Model: _____

Year: _____

Location of Title: _____

Make/Model: _____

Year: _____

Location of Title: _____

Vacation Home / Second Home:

Address: _____

Purchase price: _____

Current value: _____

Last Appraisal Date: _____

Location of Deed(s) _____

Recreational Vehicles (Boats, Trailers, Jet Skis, Snow Mobiles,

Comments: _____

_____

Furs

Comments: _____

_____

Jewelry

Comments: _____

_____

Antiques

Comments: _____

_____

Stamps

Comments: _____

_____

Coins

Comments: _____

_____

Silver & China

Comments: _____

_____

Other Assets

Comments: _____

INHERITANCE

Explain the details of any inheritance anticipated

_____

_____

_____

_____

_____

_____

_____

_____

_____

_____

_____

_____

_____

_____

_____

_____

_____

_____

DISTRIBUTION OF ASSETS*

NOTE: My will is the single best tool for delineating what items of value are to be distributed and to which individual(s). The list below is intended to serve as a backup tool. List here "Item" and name(s) of recipients. I have been as specific as possible.

How I want my furnishings, jewelry, art, divided among my loved ones:

_____

_____

_____

_____

_____

_____

_____

_____

_____

_____

▶ Make every effort to discourage arguments or disputes over personal property from wrecking family relations. Material items never take the place of love for one another.

WHERE TO LOCATE IMPORTANT PAPERS

Warning: Be cautious of writing down or giving out account numbers that may be misused by others.

Credit Cards: (Check type of card for each)

Card #1: ☐ VISA   ☐ MC   ☐ DIS   ☐ AMEX   ☐ OTHER

Name on Account: _____

Location/Comments: _____

Card #2: ☐ VISA   ☐ MC   ☐ DIS   ☐ AMEX   ☐ OTHER

Name on Account: _____

Location/Comments: _____

Card #3: ☐ VISA   ☐ MC   ☐ DIS   ☐ AMEX   ☐ OTHER

Name on Account: _____

Location/Comments: _____

Card #4: ☐ VISA   ☐ MC   ☐ DIS   ☐ AMEX   ☐ OTHER

Name on Account: _____

Location/Comments: _____

Bank Account Books:

Location/Comments: _____

_____

_____

Location/Comments: _____

_____

_____

Location/Comments: _____

_____

_____

Rental Property Payment Books:

Location/Comments: _____

_____

_____

Other Financial Records:

Location/Comments: _____

_____

_____

Location/Comments: _____

_____

_____

POWER OF ATTORNEY

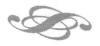

Two people with Powers of Attorney:

Name: _____

Address: _____

_____

_____

Cell #: _____

Phone #: _____

Name: _____

Address: _____

_____

_____

Cell #: _____

Phone #: _____

Comments: _____

_____

_____

_____

BIRTH CERTIFICATE & PASSPORT

BIRTH CERTIFICATE:

Two people with copies of my birth certificates:

Name: _____

Address: _____

_____

_____

Cell #: _____

Phone #: _____

Name: _____

Address: _____

_____

_____

Cell #: _____

Phone #: _____

PASSPORT:

Location: _____

ID: _____

Where Issued: _____

Date Issued: _____

Expiration Date: _____

MONTHLY BILLS & OBLIGATIONS

Name:	$ Total	Contact Phone #
Mortgage		
Homeowners Dues		
Maintenance		
Utilities		
Gas		
Water		
Electric		
Telephone		
Cable		
Internet		
Car Payment		
Insurance Premiums		
Regular Health-related		
Other		

*Make a copy, post on refrigerator and keep it current.

"EVERYONE IS NECESSARILY THE HERO OF HIS OWN STORY"

~ John Barth ~

PART V

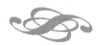

MEMORIAL PREFERENCES

This section details preferences for memorial services, locations for services, any pre-arrangements, individuals and organizations to be contacted and information to be included in an obituary .

PREFERRED FUNERAL ARRANGEMENTS

Funeral Home:

Name: _____

Phone: _____

Address: _____

I would like to be:

☐   Buried   ☐   Placed in a Mausoleum

     Location   _____

     City/State   _____

☐   Cremated

     Location   _____

     City/State   _____

     Disbursement of Ashes: _____

> **NOTE:** If any prior arrangements have been made, including prepayments, where can those documents be located, including plans for ashes if cremated?

Pre-arranged funeral plans: _____

_____

MEMORIAL PREFERENCES

I would like to be buried in (outfit preference)

    1.   _____   _____

    2.   Military uniform _____   _____

If not buried in my military uniform, I would like to wear the color(s):

_____

_____

I want these items placed in the coffin with me:

_____

_____

_____

_____

I would like this church/temple/place of worship to be used for the ceremony (name of location, city):

    Location   _____

    City/State   _____

I would like this Priest, Rabbi, or Clergyman to preside over the ceremony:

    Name: _____

    Phone: _____

    Address _____

Lodge(s) or Military Affiliation(s) to be contacted:

Name: _____

Phone: _____

Address _____

Name: _____

Phone: _____

Address _____

Name: _____

Phone: _____

Address _____

Name: _____

Phone: _____

Address _____

I would like a military honor guard or military honors at my funeral

Yes: _____

No: _____

Explain: _____

_____

_____

_____

MEMORIAL PREFERENCES

Pallbearer preferences:

Name: _____

Phone: _____

Cell Phone: _____

E-mail address: _____

Address: _____

Name: _____

Phone: _____

Cell Phone: _____

E-mail address: _____

Address: _____

Name: _____

Phone: _____

Cell Phone: _____

E-mail address: _____

Address: _____

Name: _____

Phone: _____

Cell Phone: _____

E-mail address: _____

Address: _____

I would like the following flowers:

_____

_____

_____

_____

In lieu of flowers, I would like:

_____

_____

_____

I would like the following donations made in my memory (list organizations, groups, individuals):

_____

_____

_____

I would like the following music played at the place of worship:

_____

_____

_____

I would like to have the following inscribed on my tombstone or grave marker:

_____

_____

_____

MEMORIAL PREFERENCES

I would like the following included in my obituary:

_____

_____

_____

_____

_____

_____

_____

_____

_____

_____

_____

_____

_____

_____

_____

_____

_____

_____

"IF WE CAN'T CHANGE THE INEVITABLE FUTURE, WE CAN AT LEAST PREPARE FOR IT. BY DOING THIS, WE CAN FACE THE FUTURE WITH SOME CONTROL OVER OUR DESTINY"

~ Wesley J. Smith ~

PART VI

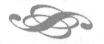

APPENDICES

LIVING WILL

A LIVING WILL IS A DOCUMENT (also known as an advanced directive) that states, prior to an illness or accident, what medical treatments you want or don't want to receive. It can also be a document in which the signer requests to be allowed to die rather than be kept alive by artificial means, if disabled beyond a reasonable expectation of recovery. When signed by a competent person, it can provide guidance for medical and healthcare decisions (such as the termination of life support or organ donation) in the event the person becomes incompetent to make such decisions.

While it is the intention of the publisher to alert users to their options in preparing for the future, please note that DC Press does not offer legal, medical or accounting advice. Prior to attempting to utilize any form presented in this book or when making an important decision effecting your future healthcare or finances, seek the advice of a legal, accounting, and/or medical professional.

A simple statement could be created and signed in front of witnesses. It is recommended that two witnesses also sign the document. Those witnesses should not be direct members of your family or someone who would benefit financially in the event of your death.

NOTE: It is very important to understand that if you fail to make a living will accessible to others, it is actually of no value and becomes completely worthless. Copies of your living will should be (1) kept with this guide and (2) given to any member of your immediate family that you feel should have one, (3) to your primary care physician and any specialists you work with, (4) your attorney, (5) and the hospital to which you feel you would most likely to taken in case of an emergency. If you are admitted to a nursing home, make sure the administration has a copy. It wouldn't be a bad idea to carry a copy in your purse or wallet.

> *Many people today are worried about the medical care they would be given if they should become terminally ill and unable to communicate. They don't want to spend months or years dependent on life-supporting machines, and they don't want to cause unnecessary emotional or financial stress for their loved ones.*
>
> **– American Hospital Association**
> "Put It In Writing: Questions and Answer or Advance Directives"

LIVING WILL DECLARATION (SAMPLE*)

THIS DECLARATION is made by _____

(Typed or printed notary name)

As I make this declaration, I am of sound mind.

I direct this declaration to my family and to anyone else who may become responsible for my health, welfare, financial, or other affairs. I hereby declare as follows:

- Should circumstances come to exist such that there is no reasonable expectation of my recovery, I direct that no extreme measures of any kind be used.

- In the event that there is a substantial question about the possibility of my recovery, or if there is no reasonable expectation of my recovery, I request that medication or other measures be utilized to reduce my physical suffering.

- I ask that this request be carried out even in the event that such measures or such medication may shorten my life.

- On behalf of my estate and myself, I hereby release from any liability all hospitals, physicians, other medical personnel, and all other individuals having any part in complying with the requests made herein above.

LIVING WILL

It is my intention that this declaration shall be valid until revoked by me.

Signed this _____ day _____ , 20 _____.

(Signature) _____

(Typed legal name) _____

Residing at: _____

This Declarant is known to me and voluntarily signed this document in my presence.

WITNESS: _____

Residing at: _____

WITNESS: _____

Residing at: _____

STATE OF_____) COUNTY OF_____)

SUBSCRIBED, SWORN TO AND ACKNOWLEDGED before me by
_____, the Declarant, and subscribed and sworn to
before me by the above-named witnesses, this _____ day of
_____, 20_____.

_____

(Notary signature)

_____

(Typed or printed notary name)

(SEAL) Notary Public for the State   _____

Residing at: _____

My commission expires: _____   (date)

Note: DC Press does not offer legal advice. Prior to attempting to
utilize any form presented in this book or when making an important
decision effecting your future healthcare or finances, seek the advice
of a legal, accounting, and/or medical professional.

DURABLE HEALTH CARE POWER OF ATTORNEY AND HEALTH CARE TREATMENT INSTRUCTIONS – LIVING WILL*

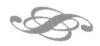

NOTE: On Making Healthcare Decisions:

You have the right to decide the type of healthcare you want. Should you be unable to make, understand, or communicate decisions about medical care, your wishes for medical treatment are most likely to be followed if you have expressed those wishes in writing in advance by:

(1)　Naming a healthcare agent to decide treatment for you; and

(2)　Giving healthcare treatment instructions to your healthcare agent or healthcare provider.

An advance healthcare directive is a written set of instructions that express your wishes for medical treatment. It may contain a

*Note: DC Press does not offer legal advice. Prior to attempting to utilize any form presented in this book or when making an important decision effecting your future healthcare or finances, seek the advice of a legal, accounting, and/or medical professional.

135

healthcare power of attorney, where you name a person called a healthcare agent to decide treatment for you, and a living will, where you tell your healthcare agent and healthcare providers your choices regarding the initiation, continuation, withholding, or withdrawal of treatment that would sustain life and other specific instructions.

You may limit your healthcare agent's involvement in deciding your medical treatment so that your healthcare agent will speak for you only when you are unable to speak for yourself or you may give your healthcare agent the power to speak for you immediately.

A living will cannot be followed unless your attending physician determines that you lack the ability to understand, make, and communicate healthcare decisions for yourself, and you are either permanently unconscious or you have an end-stage medical condition (a condition that will result in death despite the introduction or continuation of medical treatment).

You, and not your healthcare agent, remain responsible for the cost of your medical care. If you do not write down your wishes about your healthcare in advance, and if later you become unable to understand, make, or communicate these decisions, those wishes may not be honored because they may remain unknown to others.

A healthcare provider who refuses to honor your wishes about healthcare must tell you of its refusal and help to transfer you to a healthcare provider who will honor your wishes.

You should give a copy of your advance healthcare directive, living will, healthcare power of attorney or a document containing both to your healthcare agent, your physicians, family members, and others you expect would likely attend to your needs if you become unable to understand, make, or communicate decisions about medical care.

If your healthcare wishes change, tell your physician and write a new advance healthcare directive to replace your old one. It is important in selecting a healthcare agent that you choose a person you trust who is likely to be available in a medical situation where you cannot make decisions for yourself. You should inform that person that you have appointed him or her as your healthcare agent and discuss your beliefs and values with him or her so that your healthcare agent will understand your healthcare objectives.

You may wish to consult with knowledgeable, trusted individuals such as family members, your physician and/or clergy when considering an expression of your values and healthcare wishes. You are free to create your own advance healthcare directive to convey your wishes regarding medical treatment.

> **NOTE:** The form that follows is a combination of a durable power of attorney and a living will. It permits your healthcare agent the power to speak on your behalf, when you are unable to do so for yourself.

Using this form:

If you decide to use this form or create your own advance healthcare directive, you should consult with your physician and your attorney to make sure that your wishes are clearly expressed and comply with the law.

If you decide to use this form, but disagree with any of its statements, you may cross out those statements. You may add comments to this form or use your own form to help your physician or healthcare agent decide your medical care.

This form is designed to give your healthcare agent broad powers to make healthcare decisions for you, whenever you cannot make them for yourself. It is also designed to express a desire to limit or authorize care if you have an end-stage medical condition or are permanently unconscious.

If you do not desire to give your healthcare agent broad powers, or you do not wish to limit your care if you have an end-stage medical condition or are permanently unconscious, you may wish to use a different form or create your own. You should also use a different form, if you wish to express your preferences in more detail than this form allows or if you wish for your healthcare agent to be able to speak for you immediately. In these situations, it is particularly important that you consult with your attorney and physician to make sure that your wishes are clearly expressed.

This form allows you to tell your healthcare agent your goals, if you have an end-stage medical condition or other extreme and irreversible medical condition, such as advanced cancer or Alzheimer's disease. Do you want medical care applied aggressively in these situations, or would you consider such aggressive medical care burdensome and undesirable?

You may choose whether you want your healthcare agent to be bound by your instructions, or whether you want your healthcare agent to be able to decide at the time what course of treatment the healthcare agent thinks most fully reflects your wishes and values. If you are a woman and are pregnant at the time a healthcare decision would otherwise be made pursuant to this form, you need to ask about the laws of your state or commonwealth that might prohibit implementation of that decision if it directs that life-sustaining treatment, including nutrition and hydration, be withheld or withdrawn from you, unless your attending physician and an obstetrician who have examined you certify in your medical record that the life-sustaining treatment:

(1)   Will not maintain you in such a way as to permit the continuing development and live birth of the unborn child;

(2)   Will be physically harmful to you; or

(3)   Will cause pain to you that cannot be alleviated by medication.

Nevertheless investigate the specific laws that apply in your state or commonwealth where you reside.

*Note: DC Press does not offer legal advice. Prior to attempting to utilize any form presented in this book or when making an important decision effecting your future healthcare or finances, seek the advice of a legal, accounting, and/or medical professional.

DURABLE HEALTH CARE POWER OF ATTORNEY (SAMPLE)*

In town: _____ , of _____ County, _____ State, appoint the person named below to be my healthcare agent to make health and personal care decisions for me.

Effective immediately and continuously until my death or revocation by a writing signed by me or someone authorized to make healthcare treatment decisions for me, I authorize all healthcare providers or other covered entities to disclose to my healthcare agent, upon my agent's request, any information, oral or written, regarding my physical or mental health, including, but not limited to, medical and hospital records and what is otherwise private, privileged, protected or personal health information, such as health information as defined and described in the Health Insurance Portability and Accountability Act of 1996 (Public Law 104-191, 110 Stat. 1936), the regulations promulgated thereunder and any other State or local laws and rules. Information

*Note: DC Press does not offer legal advice. Prior to attempting to utilize any form presented in this book or when making an important decision effecting your future healthcare or finances, seek the advice of a legal, accounting, and/or medical professional.

disclosed by a healthcare provider or other covered entity may be re-disclosed and may no longer be subject to the privacy rules provided by 45 C.F.R. Pt. 164.

The remainder of this document will take effect when and only when I lack the ability to understand, make or communicate a choice regarding a health or personal care decision as verified by my attending physician.

MY HEALTHCARE AGENT HAS ALL OF THE FOLLOWING POWERS SUBJECT TO THE HEALTHCARE TREATMENT INSTRUCTIONS THAT FOLLOW:

(NOTE: Cross out or remove any powers you do not want to give your healthcare agent.

(1) To authorize, withhold or withdraw medical care and surgical procedures.

(2) To authorize, withhold or withdraw nutrition (food) or hydration (water) medically supplied by tube through my nose, stomach, intestines, arteries or veins.

(3) To authorize my admission to or discharge from a medical, nursing, residential or similar facility and to make agreements for my care and health insurance for my care, including hospice and/or palliative care.

(4) To hire and fire medical, social service and other support personnel responsible for my care.

(5) To take any legal action necessary to do what I have directed.

(6) To request that a physician responsible for my care issue a do-not-resuscitate (DNR) order, including an out-of-hospital DNR order, and sign any required documents and consents.

APPOINTMENT OF
HEALTH CARE AGENT
(SAMPLE)*

I appoint the following healthcare agent:

_____

(Name and relationship)

Address: _____

_____

Home Phone: _____

Cell Phone: _____

E-mail address: _____

NOTE: If you do not name a healthcare agent, healthcare providers will ask your family or an adult who knows your preferences and life values for help in determining (interpreting) your wishes for treatment.

*Note: DC Press does not offer legal advice. Prior to attempting to utilize any form presented in this book or when making an important decision effecting your future healthcare or finances, seek the advice of a legal, accounting, and/or medical professional.

NOTE: You may not appoint your doctor or other healthcare provider as your healthcare agent, unless they are related to you by blood, marriage or adoption

If my healthcare agent is not readily available or if my healthcare agent is my spouse and an action for divorce is filed by either of us after the date of this document, I appoint the person or persons named below in the order named. (Note: It can be helpful, but not required, to name alternative healthcare agents.)

First Alternative Healthcare Agent:

_____

(Name and relationship)

Address: _____

_____

Home Phone: _____

Cell Phone: _____

E-mail address: _____

Second Alternative Healthcare Agent:

_____

(Name and relationship)

Address: _____

_____

Home Phone: _____

Cell Phone: _____

E-mail address: _____

"IF YOU LOOK INSIDE YOURSELF, AND YOU BELIEVE, YOU CAN BE YOUR OWN HERO"

~ Mariah Carey ~

Notes

The following space is provided for individuals to add all of the "extra information" that hasn't been presented in other parts of this guide - or to embellish things said earlier but requiring additional space. Anything goes here. Feel free to give future caregivers more insight into the real you.

Notes

Notes

Notes

Notes

Notes

"WE'RE SO ENGAGED IN DOING THINGS TO ACHIEVE PURPOSES OF OUTER VALUE THAT WE FORGET THE INNER VALUE, THE RAPTURE THAT IS ASSOCIATED WITH BEING ALIVE."

~ Joseph Campbell ~

INTERNET RESOURCES

These resources are recommended for your consideration and review. It is your personal responsibility to stay educated and on top of key issues that are or will be impacting your life.

This list has resources in a number of key areas, but we encourage you to add to it as you discover new sites that may be useful to you. Please keep in mind that this is a very useful tool in addressing issues of importance to you and your family.

AARP
General Information: *www.aarp.org*
Independent Living: *www.aarp.org/family/caregiving*
Taxes: *www.aarp.org/taxaide*
Public Benefits Outreach Program: *www.aarp.org/money/lowincomehelp*

AMA (American Medical Association)
www.ama-assn.org

AMA Doctor Finder
http://webapps.ama-assn.org/doctorfinder/home.html

CancerCare
www.cancercare.org

Cancer Caregiving
www.cancercaregiving.com

Cancer.net (American Society of Clinical Oncology)
Home: *www.asco.org*
Caregiving: *www.asco.org/patient/Coping/Caregiving*

Caregiver's Home Companion
www.caregivershome.com

Caregiving.com
www.caregiving.com

Caring.com
www.caring.com

Caring Connections
www.caringinfo.org/caringforsomeone

Compare Hospitals
www.hospitalcompare.hhs.gov

Complaints
*www.healthfinder.gov/scripts/SearchContext.asp?topic=14309&Branch
=3*

Elder Care Locator
www.eldercare.gov/Eldercare/Public/Home.asp

Family Caregiving 101
www.familycaregiving101.org

Family Caregiver Alliance
www.caregiver.org/caregiver/jsp/home.jsp

Find a Facility
www.healthfinder.gov/scripts/Topics.asp?context=8&keyword=147&Branch=3

Funeral and Burial Planning:
There is an objective article on the subject at:
http://dying.about.com/od/funeralsandmemorials/ht/plan_a_funeral.htm

Healthcare Quality
www.ahrq.gov/consumer/guidetoq

Healthy Aging (Centers for Disease Control)
www.cdc.gov/aging/caregiving/index.htm

Heart of Caregiving
www.americanheart.org/presenter.jhtml?identifier=3039829

Health Insurance
www.healthinsuranceinfo.net

HIPAA
www.healthfinder.gov/scripts/SearchContext.asp?topic=5706&Branch=3

Hospice
www.hospicenet.org
www.nhpco.org/custom/directory/main.cfm

Long-Term Care
www.longtermcareliving.com

Lotsa Helping Hands
www.lotsahelpinghands.com

Managed Care
www.pohly.com/terms.html

Mayo Clinic
www.mayoclinic.com
www.mayoclinic.com/health/alzheimers/AZ00013

Medicare
Home: *www.medicare.gov*
Medicare Health Plans:
www.medicare.gov/MPPF/Include/DataSection/Questions/Welcome.asp

Medication Errors
www.fda.gov/cder/drug/mederrors/default.htm

MedicineNet.com
www.medicinenet.com/caregiving/article.htm

MedlinePlus (National Institutes of Health)
Www.nlm.nih.gov/medlineplus/caregivers.html

Military Sites:

> **Official Military Sites:**
> Airforce Official Site: *http://www.af.mil/*
> Army Official Site: *http://www.army.mil/*
> Navy Official Site: *http://www.navy.mil*
> Marines Official Site: *http://www.marines.mil*
> Coast Guard Official Site: *http://www.uscg.mil*

Military Sites - continued:

Official Military Relief Funds:
Air Force Aid Society: *http://www.afas.org/*
Army Emergency Relief: *http://www.aerhq.org/*
Navy-Marine Corps Relief Society: *http://www.nmcrs.org/*
National Veterans Foundation: *http://www.nvf.org/*
PTSD Counseling, VA benefits advocacy, food, shelter, employment training,
 legal aid, or suicide intervention

Benfits Claims / Legal:
National Veterans Legal Services Program: *http://www.nvlsp.org/*
U.S. Court of Appeals for Veteran Claims: *http://www.uscourts.cavc.gov/*
U.S. Dept. of Veterans Affairs: *http://www.va.gov/*
Veterans Consortium Pro Bono Program: *http://www.vetsprobono.org/*
(Free attorneys for pending appeals for veterans claims)

Employment:
Career One Stop: *http://www.careeronestop.org/MilitaryTransition/*
(Sponsored by U. S. Dept. of Labor)
Employment Support of the Guard and Reserve: *http://esgr.org/site/*
National Veterans Employment Program: *http://www1.va.gov/Nvep/*
(Part of U.S. Dept. of Veterans Affairs)
Vet Success: *http://www.vetsuccess.gov/* (Part of U.S. Dept. of Veterans Affairs)
Veterans Employment Coordination Service: *http://www4.va.gov/vecs/*
(Part of U.S. Dept. of Veterans Affairs)

Shelter
National Coalition for Homeless Veterans: *http://www.nchv.org/*
United States Veterans Initiative: *http://www.usvetsinc.org/*

Spouse, Family & Parenting:
Army Wife Network: *http://www.ArmyWifeNetwork.com/*
Blue Star Mothers of America, Inc.:
*http://www.bluestarmothers.org/mc/page.do?sitePageId=59966&orgId=bs
ma*
Michigan Military Moms: *http://www.michiganmilitarymoms.org/*
Military.com: http://www.military.com/opinion/0,15202,140604,00.html
Military Parents Alliance: http://www.militaryparents.org/
Military Parent Support & Information:
http://childparenting.about.com/cs/parentsupport/a/militaryparent2.htm
Military Moms: http://www.militarymoms.net/
Mothers of Military Support: http://www.mothersofmilitarysupport.com/
Mothers of the Military: http://www.mothersofthemilitary.org/home.html
Operation Military Parents: http://www.operationmilitaryparents.com/
Proud Army Moms: http://www.proudarmymoms.org/
The Military Family Network: http://www.emilitary.org/parents1.html
Type-A Mom: http://www.typeamom.net/mom-types/military-moms.html

Military Sites - continued:

Stress Management/Counseling:
Military One Source: *http://www.militaryonesource.com/*
(Resource for active duty personnel and families)
Soldiers Project: *http://www.thesoldiersproject.org/*

Veterans Organizations:
American Legion: *http://www.legion.org/*
American Veterans: *http://www.amvets.org/*
Disabled American Veterans: *http://www.dav.org/veterans/MilitaryAffairs.aspx*
http://www.dav.org/veterans/veteransaffairs.aspx
GI Bill *http://www.legion.org/mygibill*
Iraq and Afghanistan Veterans of America: *http://iava.org/index.php*
Military Officers Association of America: *http://www.msc@moaa.org*
http://www.purpleheart.org
National Veterans Foundation: *http://www.nvf.org/*
Paralyzed Veterans of America:
http://www.pva.org/site/PageServer?pagename=homepage
Veterans of Foreign Wars *http://www.vfw.org/*
Wounded Warrior Project *http://www.woundedwarriorproject.org/*
Military Order of the Purple Heart of the U.S.A., Inc.:

My Care Community
www.mycarecommunity.org

National Alliance for Caregivers
www.caregiving.org

National Association for Home Care and Hospice
www.nahc.org

National Caregiving Association
www.caregivingfoundation.org

National Family Caregivers Association
www.nfcacares.org

National Family Caregiver Support Program (Dept. of Health and Human Services)
www.aoa.gov/prof/aoaprog/caregiver/careprof/progguidance/resources/caregiving_terms.aspx

Quality Care Connections
(Rosalynn Carter Institute for Caregiving and Johnson & Johnson)
www.qualitycareconnections.org/QCC/Welcome.html

Patient Records Confidentiality
www.ama-assn.org/ama/pub/category/4610.html

Power of Attorney
http://www.uslegalforms.com/poweratty.htm

Prevention Magazine
www.prevention.com/cda/homepage.do

Privacy
www.ama-assn.org/ama/pub/category/4610.html

Privacy Myths
www.myphr.com/rights/common_myths.asp

Rosalynn Carter Institute for Caregiving
www.rosalynncarter.org/
www.qualitycareconnections.org/QCC/Welcome.html

Social Security
http://www.ssa.gov/

Strength for Caring (sponsored by Johnson & Johnson)
www.strengthforcaring.com/
RESO

Suite 101
www.suite101.com/welcome.cfm/elderly_caregiving

Support Groups
www.healthfinder.gov/scripts/SearchContext.asp?topic=833&Branch=3

The Center for Volunteer Caregiving
www.volunteercaregiving.org

Third Age
www.thirdage.com/caregiving

Understand Your Medications
www.usp.org/pdf/EN/patientSafety/justAskDozenQs.pdf

Veterans Benefits
Military Records Request: *http://www.archives.gov*
National Cemetery Administration: *http://www.cem.va.gov/*
VA Facility Directory: *http://www1.va.gov*
Veterans Health Administration: *http://www.appc1.va.gov*
Veterans Benefits Administration: *http://www.va.gov/*
Federal Benefits For Veterans:
http://www1.va.gov/opa/vadocs/Fedben.pdf

Visiting Nurse Association
http://vnaa.org/vnaa/gen/HTML~Home.aspx
Finding a visiting nurse in your area:
http://www.vnaa.org/vnaa/Searches/findvna.aspx

WebMD
www.webmd.com/healthy-aging/caregiving-insights/default.htm

Well Spouse Association
www.wellspouse.org

Wiser Women Institute for a Secure Retirement
*www.wiserwomen.org/portal/index.php?option=com_frontpage&Itemid
=1*

THIS BOOK IS 'LOVE INSURANCE' FOR YOUR FAMILY. THE PREMIUMS ARE LOW, BUT THE DIVIDENDS ARE PRICELESS!

~ Dee Marrella ~

WORDS & PHRASES TO KEEP HANDY

On the following pages, you have been provided with the major terms that are being used in newspapers, magazines, on TV and the radio when discussing issues impacting Americans at the time of publication. The author and publisher believe these are important words and phrases with which you should become familiar and conversant. Should you find that some of these words become very much a part of your life, you might improve your understanding by reading up on them by visiting the library near your home and by making use of the wide array of information available on the Internet.

▶ **NOTE:** DC Press does not offer legal advice. Prior to attempting to utilize any form presented in this book or when making an important decision effecting your future healthcare or finances, seek the advice of legal, accounting and/or medical professionals.

A

Acute Care

Special care that is provided typically for a brief period of time to treat a certain illness or condition. This type of care often includes short-term hospital stays, doctor's visits, surgery, and X-rays.

Adult Care Home

A residence that offers services of a housing and personal care nature for 3 up to 16 residents. The owner or manager usually provides services such as meals, supervision, and transportation. Can also be known as a board and care home or group home.

Advanced Directive for Health Care

Legal document, such as a living will, a durable power of attorney for health-care, or both), prepared ahead of time and signed by a living and competent person in order to provide guidance for medical and healthcare decisions (including the termination of life support and organ donation) in the event that he or she becomes incompetent to make such decisions.

Alzheimer's Disease

A progressive, irreversible disease of unknown cause that is the most common form of dementia, marked by the loss of cognitive ability (due to degeneration of the brain cells and subsequent loss of memory). It usually starts in late middle age or in old age as a loss of memory of recent events, which spreads to memories for more distant events. It progresses on average over the course of five to ten or fifteen years to a profound intellectual decline characterized by dementia and personal helplessness.

Assisted Living Facility

Often licensed and known as residential care facilities or rest homes, a residence that combines housing, supportive services, personalized assistance and healthcare designed to meet the individual's needs on a daily basis emphasizing residents' privacy and choice. These needs may include bathing, dressing, balancing a checkbook, medication reminders, and/or housework for example. In many assisted living facilities, 24-hour supportive services are available to meet the planned and unplanned needs of the residents. These settings in which services are delivered may include self-contained apartment units or single or shared room units with private or area baths. Assisted Living Facilities can be similar to a Board and Care Home, but are typically larger.

Assistive Devices

A range of products designed to help elders or people with disabilities lead more independent lives. Examples include walking aids, motorized wheelchairs, lifts, raised/elevated toilet seats, bathtub seats, ramps, and handrails for example. In some cases, modifications to the living facility are required in order to properly utilize the devices. Also known as Architectural Adaptations, these are structural fabrications or remodeling in the home, work site, or other areas (including for example ramps, lifts, lighting, kitchen remodeling, bathroom adaptations) that remove or reduce physical barriers for an individual with a disability.

B

Beneficiary

A person or entity (perhaps a charity or estate) that receives a benefit or proceeds from something, a person or entity named or otherwise entitled to receive the proceeds (principal or income or both) from a will, trust, insurance policy, retirement plan, annuity or other contract. An individual covered by Medicare is also called a beneficiary.

Benefit Trigger

Before benefits are paid, certain benefit triggers and other conditions must be met. A benefit trigger is usually met by measuring a person's ability to do one or more activities of daily living(ADLs), such as bathing or dressing, or by testing the person's cognitive abilities. Also, it is a condition that must exist in order for an insurance company to pay benefits under a long-term care insurance policy. Benefits are triggered for nursing home care, assisted living, or home care when a person can't do two of the ADLs listed in the policy, or when a person has an obvious cognitive impairment like Alzheimer's and has met other conditions in the policy. Tax-qualified policies use a list of six ADLs: Bathing, Dressing, Transferring, Eating, Toileting, and Continence Non-tax qualified policies use seven ADLs, adding ambulating (walking) to the list.

Benefits

A monetary sum or payment made or an entitlement available in accordance with an insurance policy or a public assistance program, or to someone else, such as a health care provider, to whom the insured person has assigned the benefits.

Board and Care Home

A Board and Care Home usually offers seniors supervision and some personal care (such as meals and transportation), but few onsite medical services. A small number of residents live (between 3 and 16) in a group home, sometimes in a refurbished single-family home. A Board and Care Home can be the same as an Assisted Living Facility, but on a smaller scale.

C

Care/Case Management

Care management is a coordinated care function (single point of entry) incorporating case finding, assessment, care planning, negotiation, care plan implementation, monitoring, and advocacy to assist clients and their families with complex needs in obtaining appropriate services. This program(operated privately or through social service agencies or public programs) locates, mobilizes and manages a variety of home care and other services needed by a frail elderly person at risk of nursing home placement. An assessment is performed to identify needs, and appropriate services are secured to enable the individual to remain at home. Case managers assist in gaining access to needed services for those persons eligible. They monitor the provision of these services as well as initiate and oversee the assessment and reassessment of an individual's level and plan of care.

Care Manager

A health care professional, typically a nurse or social worker, who arranges, monitors, or coordinates long-term care services. A care manager may also assess a patient's needs and develop a plan of care, subject to approval by the patient's physician. They may also be referred to as a care coordinator or case manager.

Chore Services

In short, they are assistance with chores such as home repairs, yard work, and heavy housecleaning. They are non-continuous household maintenance tasks intended to increase the safety of the individual(s) in their residence(s).

Typically these tasks are limited to the following: replacing light bulbs, fuses, electric plugs and frayed cords, door locks, window catches, water pipes, faucets and/or washers. They can include installation and repair of safety equipment, screens and storm windows, weather stripping around doors, window shades and curtain rods. Furniture repair, the cleaning of appliances, rugs, basements and attics to remove potential hazards are included as are washing walls and windows, scrubbing floors, pest control, mowing grass and raking leaves, clearing ice, snow, and leaves from sidewalks, driveways, and step, and trimming overhanging branches.

Chronically Ill Individual

A chronically ill individual, as defined by the federal government, is someone who has been certified (at least in the past twelve months) by a licensed health care practitioner as (1) Being unable to perform, without substantial assistance from another individual, at least two daily living activities (eating, toileting, transferring, bathing, dressing, and continence) for at least 90 days due to a loss of functional capacity or (2) Requiring substantial supervision to protect the individual from threats to health and safety due to severe cognitive impairment.

Chronic Illness or Condition

There are two types of illnesses: acute and chronic. Acute illnesses (like a cold or the flu) are usually over relatively quickly. Chronic illnesses, though, are long-lasting health conditions (the word "chronic" comes from the Greek word chronos, meaning time). An illness or other condition with one or more of the following characteristics: permanency, residual disability, requires rehabilitation training, or requires a long period of supervision, observation, or care. Typically, it is a disease or condition that lasts over a long period of time and cannot be cured; it is often associated with disability.

Codicil

A supplement, appendix, or legal change to will.

Congregate Housing

Congregate (or supported) housing is a group housing option (such as individual apartments) for the elderly and disabled, with private living quarters and common dining and social areas with additional safety measures such as emergency call buttons. Support services vary, but usually include meals, housekeeping and activities. People living in a congregate housing facility require little or no personal care assistance.

Continuing Care Retirement Community (CCRC)

A privately owned retirement community for people who cannot or who prefer not to maintain an independent household because they need some kind of long-term assistance or medical care that offer a broad range of services and degrees or levels of care based on individual needs. Also known as life care, these communities can range from full-time care in nursing homes to assisted living to independent living situations. It is not unusual for continuing care retirement communities (CCRCs) to be expensive and entry fees or payments required prior to acceptance along with continuing monthly fees.

Custodial Care

Room and board in a nursing home where assistance with activities of daily living is provided such as bathing, dressing, eating, and other non-medical care that most people do themselves. Medicare does not pay for custodial care. Medicaid provides the majority of reimbursement for custodial care, although very little. It is important to note that it is typical that individuals without professional training may provide this type of care.

D

Depression

Depression is an illness that affects both mind and body— one that can make it difficult to handle everyday life. It is one of the most undiagnosed conditions among seniors. Research has linked depression to an imbalance in two of the naturally occurring chemicals in the brain and body, serotonin and norepinephrine. These chemicals help regulate how your body perceives thoughts and feelings including pain. While people with a family history of depression may be more prone to the disease, anyone can become depressed. Sometimes the triggers are external – for example, relationship troubles or financial problems; at other times the disease can be brought about by physical illness or hormonal shifts. Depression can also occur without any identifiable trigger at all. Symptoms can include a persistent sad, anxious or "empty"mood, loss of interest or pleasure in activities once enjoyed and difficulty sleeping.

Discharge Planner

A healthcare professional or social worker who assists hospital patients and their families in transitioning from the hospital to another level of care such as a rehabilitation center, rehabilitation in a skilled nursing facility, home health care in the patient's home, or long-term care in a nursing home.

Do Not Resuscitate Order

A code or order usually appearing in a patient's medical record indicating that in the event the heart and/or breathing stops, no intervention be undertaken by staff. Death occurs undisturbed. This does not mean that the individual does not receive care. Continuing care is provided as it would to any individual (medications for pain, antibiotics, etc.) except as stated above.

Durable Medical Equipment

Known as DME (also known as Home Medical Equipment), this is equipment that: can be used over and over again, is ordinarily used for medical purposes, and is generally not useful to a person who isn't sick, injured or disabled. Initially, it is medical equipment ordered by a doctor who writes a prescription for it for use in the home. Equipment includes canes, crutches, walkers, hospital beds, wheelchairs, lifts, and prosthetics used at home. DME may be covered by Medicaid and in part by Medicare or private insurance.

E

Elder Care

A specialty in legal practice, covering estate planning, wills, trusts, arrangements for care, social security and retirement benefits, protection against elder abuse (physical, emotional and financial), and other concerns of older people.

Estate

The whole of one's possessions, especially all the property and debts left by one at death.

Executor

The person or institution appointed by a court or testator to execute his will, or to see its provisions carried into effect after his decease.

F

Fiduciary

A person, such as a trustee or guardian, who holds assets of another person or beneficiary, often with the legal authority and duty to make decisions regarding financial matters on behalf of the other party. It is illegal for a fiduciary to misappropriate money for personal gain.

Family Medical Leave Act

Known as FMLA, the Federal law that requires any firm with over 50 employees to grant an eligible employee up to a total of 12 work weeks of unpaid leave during any 12-month period to care for a family member with a serious health condition such as a senior. The employer must maintain an employee's group health insurance benefits while taking FMLA leave and must reinstate the employee in the same job upon returning from FMLA leave.

G

Guardian

One who is legally responsible (appointed by a court) for the care and management of the person or property of an individual who is unable to take care of himself or herself.

H

Health Maintenance Organization

Known as an HMO, group insurance that entitles members to services of participating hospitals, clinics and physicians. For those aged 65 and older, a type of Medicare managed care plan where a group of doctors, hospitals and other health care providers agree to give healthcare to Medicare beneficiaries for a pre-established amount of money from Medicare every month. Typically members must get all of their care from the providers who participate in the plan. Use of providers outside the HMO, will require payment out of pocket for services.

Heir

Someone who inherits assets from an estate of another person who has died. The heir does not have to pay income tax or estate tax on the value of the inheritance received.

Home Care

Caring for an aging or impaired person in their home by providing homemaking, meal preparation, shopping, transportation and assistance with activities of daily living.

Home Care Aides

Individuals who provide non-mechanical assistance to impaired individuals in their homes. Also known as domiciliary care, is health care or supportive care provided in the patient's home by healthcare professionals, often referred to as home health care or formal care. In the United States, it is also known as skilled care. Such care can also be provided by family and friends, also known as caregivers, primary caregiver, or voluntary caregivers who give informal care. Often, the term home care is used to distinguish non-medical care or custodial care, which is care that is provided by persons who are not nurses, doctors, or other licensed medical personnel, whereas the term home healthcare, refers to care that is provided by licensed personnel.

Home Health Agency (HHA)

Also known as an HHA, this is a public or private operation providing home health services which are supervised by a licensed health professional in the patient's home either directly or through arrangements with other organizations.

Home Health Care

Generally, home health services are initiated when an individual is no longer able to care for him or herself due to serious changes in their health. It is not unusual for a doctor, nurse, hospital discharge planner or case manager to suggest that professional help in the home, as an alternative to hospitalization or a nursing home, to assist with health care needs on around-the-clock basis – although home healthcare services are usually provided on a visit basis rather than an hourly basis. Readmission to a hospital can often be prevented or delayed. Most services must be ordered by a physician, and must be medically necessary to maintain or improve your health condition, in order to be covered by health insurance. Home healthcare services are usually provided on a visit basis rather than an hourly basis.

Homebound

An individual is understood to be homebound if absences from the home are infrequent or of relatively short duration, or are attributable to the need to receive medical treatment. Leaving home to receive medical treatment includes going to adult daycare so long as the individual receives therapeutic, psycho-social or medical treatment from a licensed or state-certified adult day-care facility. Any absence for a religious service is considered an absence of short duration and doesn't negate the homebound status.

Hospice and Hospice Care

This is a program providing palliative care that improves the quality of life of patients facing terminal illness (end-of-life) and their families. The prevention and relief of suffering by means of early identification and impeccable assessment and treatment of pain and other problems, physical, psycho-social and spiritual is all part of the program. Hospices 1) provide relief from pain and other distressing symptoms, 2) affirm life and regard dying as a normal process, 3) neither hasten or postpone death intentionally, 4) integrate both psychological and spiritual aspects of patient care, 5) offer a support system to help patients live as actively as possible until death, 6) offer a support system to help the family cope during the patient's illness and through bereavement, 7) use a team approach to address the needs of patients and their families, including bereavement counseling, when needed, (8) are designed to enhance quality of life, and may also positively influence the course of an illness, and 9) are applicable early in the course of illness, in conjunction with other therapies that are intended to prolong life, such as radiation or chemotherapy, and includes those investigations needed to better understand and manage distressing clinical complications. Hospice care can be provided at home, in a facility with a homelike setting, a hospital or a nursing home. The care includes physical care, counseling and support services, but does not attempt to cure any illness.

I

Independent Living Facility

A type of living arrangement in which personal care services such as meals, housekeeping, transportation, and assistance with activities of daily living are available as needed to people who still live on their own in a residential facility. In most cases, the "assisted living" residents pay a regular monthly rent. They typically pay additional fees for the services they get.

Instrumental Activities of Daily Living

Instrumental activities of daily living (also known as IADLs) are activities related to independent living (without the assistance or substantial supervision of another person) and include for example grocery shopping and preparing meals, managing money, shopping for groceries or personal items, performing light or heavy housework, doing laundry, using a telephone, paying bills, and taking daily medications. Most long-term care insurance policies will not pay benefits for the loss of ability to perform IADLs.

Intermediate Care

Needed for people in stable condition who require daily care, but not round-the-clock nursing supervision. Typically ordered by a doctor and supervised by registered nurses. Intermediate care is less specialized than skilled nursing care and it usually involves more personal care. Intermediate care is generally needed for a long period of time.

Intermediate Care Facility

Nursing homes most frequently come to mind when people envision what is in reality an intermediate care facility (also known as an ICF). Recognized under the Medicaid program, they provide health-related care and services to individuals who do not require acute or skilled nursing care, but who, because of their mental or physical condition, require care and services above the level of room and board available only through facility placement. These facilities often have more mobile, less acutely ill residents than a skilled nursing facility, which provides sophisticated medical care to people with acute medical needs. An ICF is staffed by a team of nurses under the supervision of an attending physician. Much of the care provided in an ICF—often called "custodial" or "maintenance care" and provided in large part by nurses' aides—is personal care like help with bathing, dressing, and eating. An ICF is often set up as a wing of a skilled nursing facility. Specific requirements for ICF's vary by state. Institutions for care of the mentally retarded or people with related conditions (ICF/MR) are also included. The distinction between "health-related care and services" and "room and board" is important since ICF's are subject to different regulations and coverage requirements than institutions that do not provide health-related care and services.

J

Joint Tenant with Right of Survivorship

Ownership of property by two or more people in which the survivors automatically gain ownership of a descendent's interest. Upon the death of any joint tenant, his or her ownership interest automatically passes to the surviving joint tenant.

L

Level of Care

Known as LOC, an assessment of the type of care necessary to meet the individual needs of the client and their eligibility for programs and services. The assessment takes into consideration the client's needs in all aspects of development, level of functioning (levels include: protective, intermediate, and skilled), and potential to benefit from a particular program.

Life Care Plan

Specific plan developed by a professional known as a Life Care Planner.An important tool in the future of a catastrophically injured person (suchas on the job, in a serious accident, through medical malpractice). The Life Care Planner summarizes the medical, educational, vocational, psycho-social, and daily living needs of the individual who can function indefinitely only with professional assistance. The Life Care Planner projects the long-term costs of care, and establishes rehabilitative goals while coordinating future care providers in order to best assure a continued recovery.

Living Trust

A trust created for and individual (the trustor) and administered by another party during the trustor's lifetime. The living trust may be formed because the trustor is either incapable of managing or unwilling to manage his or her assets. The trust can be revocable or irrevocable, depending upon the trustor's wishes. It avoids probate and assets are distributed typically faster than through a will. Also called an inter vivos trust.

Living Will

A legal document (a will) in which the signer requests not to be kept alive by medical life-support systems in the event of a terminal illness or incapacity.

Long-Term Care

Term used to represent a range of services that address the health, social, and personal care needs of individuals delivered over a long period of time to persons who have never developed or have lost some capacity for self care.

Long-Term Care Insurance

Long-term care insurance (LTC or LTCI), an insurance product sold in the United States, helps provide for the cost of long-term care beyond a predetermined period, and designed to provide coverage for necessary medical or personal care services provided outside of a hospital setting. Long-term care insurance covers care generally not covered by health insurance, Medicare, or Medicaid. It provides for skilled, intermediate, and custodial care in a private home, adult daycare setting, assisted-living facility, and/or nursing home.

M

Managed Care

A system of healthcare that combines delivery and payment; and influences utilization of services, by employing management techniques designed to promote the delivery of cost-effective healthcare. Organizations created included MNOs, PPOs, and PSOs. Members pay a pre-established monthly amount for care to be provided regardless of the amount required.

Medical Power of Attorney

An advance directive with written instructions that appoint someone to make decisions about an individual's medical care.

N

Nursing Home

Filling a special niche in health care, a private facility that provides living quarters and care for the elderly or the chronically ill who do not need the intensive, acute care of a hospital but for whom remaining home is no longer appropriate. Licensed by the state, it offers residents personal care as well as skilled nursing care on a 24-hour basis. Nursing homes are capable of caring for individuals with a wide range of medical conditions. Provides nursing care, personal care, room and board, supervision, medication, therapies and rehabilitation.

Nursing homes come in different sizes and with different names. They may also be known as: health centers, havens or manors, homes for the aged, nursing homes or centers, care centers, continuing care centers, living centers, or convalescent centers.

Nurse Practitioner

Known as an NP, a registered nurse working in an expanded nursing role, usually with a focus on meeting primary healthcare needs. They conduct physical examinations, interpret laboratory results, select plans of treatment, identify medication requirements, and perform certain medical management activities for selected health conditions. Some specialize in geriatric care.

O

Ombudsman

A representative who investigates complaints and mediates fair settlements for a public agency or a private nonprofit, especially between aggrieved parties such as older consumers who reside in long-term care facilities and the facility, institution or organization.

Outpatient

A patient who does not reside in or has not been admitted to the hospital where they are being treated and receiving ambulatory care.

P

Personal Emergency Response System

In case of a fall or other medical emergency, an electronic device enables the user to contact assistance 24-hours a day simply by pressing a button in the event of an emergency (personal medical issue, a fall, fire, etc.)

Physician Assistant

A specially trained and licensed or otherwise credentialed individual who performs tasks under the direction of a supervising physician which might otherwise be performed by a physician. Usually called a PA.

Plan of Care

A written plan describing what specific services and care needed for an individual's health problem. An individual's plan of care must be prepared or approved by their doctor.

Point of Service Plan

A health plan that allows members to choose to receive services from a participating or non-participating network provider, usually with a financial disincentive for going outside the network. More of a product than an organization, POS plans can be offered by HMOs, PPOs, or self-insured employers.

Power of Attorney

A General Power of Attorney is a legal document which gives the person you choose (the agent) the power to manage your assets and financial affairs while you are alive. The simplest and least expensive legal device for authorizing a person to manage the affairs of another. The document must be signed by an individual (the principal) while that person has the required legal capacity to give their agent clear and concise instructions. The appointment may be for a fixed period and can be revoked by the individual at any time providing he or she still has the legal capacity to do so. A power of attorney ceases when the individual dies. The executor named in your will then takes over the responsibilities of your estate.

A Durable Power of Attorney stays valid even if you become unable to handle your own affairs (incapacitated). If you don't specify that you want your power of attorney to be durable, it will automatically end if you later become incapacitated.

A Limited Power of Attorney allows the principal to give only specific powers to the agent. The limited power of attorney is used to allow the agent to handle specific matters when the principal is unavailable or unable to do so. Forms needed for specific states maybe found at: Http://www.uslegal-forms.com/poweratty.htm.

Power of Attorney for Health Care

Allows an individual to appoint a person to make medical decisions for them in the event they are unable to do so for themselves. A written legal document in which one person (the principal) appoints another person To make healthcare decisions on behalf of the principal in the event the principal becomes incapacitated (the document defines incapacitation). This instrument can contain instructions about specific medical treatment that should be applied or withheld. While its purpose remains essentially the same from state to state, the name of this document can vary; for example, in Florida it is called a Designation of Health Care Surrogate. Forms needed for specific states maybe found at: http://www.uslegal-forms.com/poweratty.htm.

Preferred Provider Organization

A type of managed care plan (known as a PPO). Members have a choice of utilizing healthcare providers in the PPO network, or hospitals, doctors and other healthcare professionals outside the plan for an additional cost.

Primary Care Physician

Physician responsible for a person's general or basic health care (known as General Practitioner or Family Doctor). The physician an individual sees first for most health problems. They make sure you get the care needed to stay healthy. They might talk with other more specialized doctors and healthcare providers and make a referral to them. In many Medicare managed care plans, participants must see their primary care doctor before seeing other healthcare providers.

Primary Caregiver

The individual or individuals, usually the spouse or adult child, over the age of eighteen years designated by a qualified patient who has consistently assumed responsibility for the housing, health or safety of that qualified patient on a day-by-day basis. They take responsibility for caring for the physical, psychological and social needs of another individual.

Probate

Proof that a will is valid and that its terms are being carried out. Probate is accomplished by an executor/ executrix (if a will exists) who is paid a fee based on the size of the estate that passes through the will. Certain trusts and jointly owned property pass to beneficiaries without being subject to probate and the attendant fee. Executor or a court-appointed administrator (if there is no will), manages and distributes a decedent's property to heirs and/or beneficiaries.

Provider

A person or organization who helps in identifying or preventing or treating illness and/or disability.

These can be any of the following: a properly-licensed doctor, healthcare professional, hospital, or other healthcare facility, including a home health agency, that provides healthcare or related social services.

Provider Sponsored Organization

Similar to an HMO or Medicare HMO except that this managed care organization (known as a PSO) is owned by the providers in that plan and these providers share the financial risk assumed by the organization.

R

Rehabilitation Services

Services designed to improve/restore a person's functioning; includes physical therapy, occupational therapy, and/orspeech therapy. May be provided at home or in long-term care facilities. May be covered in part by Medicare. Because rehabilitation services are an optional Medicaid benefit, not all states provide this service.

Residential Care

Room, board and personal care provided in a fashion that falls between the nursing care delivered in skilled and intermediate care facilities and the assistance provided through social services. Typically 24-hour supervision is provided to individuals requiring assistance with daily living activities

Residential Care Facility

Generic term for group homes, specialized apartment complexes, or other institutions providing care services (room, board and personal care) for residents. The term is used to refer to a range of residential care options including assisted living facilities, board and care homes and skilled nursing facilities providing 24-hour supervision of individuals who, because of old age or impairments, necessarily need assistance with the activities of daily living.

Respite

The in-home care of chronically ill beneficiary intended to give the caregiver a rest. Can also be provided by a hospice or a nursing facility.

S

Skilled Care

Institutional care (a subset of post-acute care) that is less intensive than hospital care in its nursing and medical service, but which includes procedures whose administration requires the training and skills of an RN. This care is usually needed 24 hours a day, must be ordered by a physician, and must follow a plan of care. Individuals usually get skilled care in a nursing home but may also receive it in other places. "Higher level" of care (such as injections, catheterizations, and dressing changes) provided by trained medical professionals, including nurses, doctors, and physical therapist. Both Medicare and Medicaid reimburse for care at the skilled level. Medicare reimburses 100 days of skilled care following an acute hospitalization. This is commonly available in designated beds in a nursing home.

Skilled Nursing Care

Skilled care that is administered or supervised by Registered Nurses. Skilled nursing care can include: intravenous injections, tube feeding, and changing sterile dressings on a wound. Any service that could be safely done by an average non-medical person without the supervision of a Registered Nurse is not considered skilled care.

Skilled Nursing Facility

Also known as nursing homes, convalescent hospitals and/or rest homes, SNFs provide continuous (24-hour) nursing services (care and rehabilitation in addition to regular medical services) under a registered nurse or licensed vocational nurse. They are equipped to provide more extensive care needs, such as administering injections, monitoring blood pressure, and caring for patients on ventilators, or those requiring intravenous feeding. However, many residents in skilled nursing facilities may be receiving only"custodial" care such as help with bathing, eating, getting in and out of bed, and using the toilet. In addition, SNFs must provide recreational activities for residents. They may also provide rehabilitative services, such as physical, occupational, or speech therapies. SNF care can be costly (an average of $40,000 per year).

Special Health Maintenance Organization

Known as SHMO, this organization provides a unique alternative to traditional HMO by combining preventive, acute and long-term care benefits. A managed system of health and long-term care services geared toward an elderly client population. Under this model, a single provider entity assumes responsibility for a full range of acute inpatient, ambulatory, rehabilitative, extended home health and personal care services under a fixed budget, which is determined prospectively. Elderly people who reside in the target service area are voluntarily enrolled. Once enrolled, individuals are obligated to receive all SHMO covered services through SHMO providers, similar to the operation of a medical model health maintenance organization.

Social Security Disability Insurance

A system (known as SSDI) of federally provided payments to eligible workers (and, in some cases, their families) when they are unable to continue working because of a disability. Benefits begin with the sixth full month of disability and continue until the individual is capable of substantial gainful activity.

Special Care Units

Designated area of a residential care facility or nursing home that cares specifically for the needs of people with Alzheimer's, head injuries, dementia, or other specific disorders.

Spend Down

Under the Medicaid program, a method by which an individual establishes Medicaid eligibility by reducing gross income through incurring medical expenses until net income (after medical expenses) meets Medicaid financial requirements. A resident spends down when he/she is no longer sufficiently covered by a third-party payer (usually Medicare) and has exhausted all personal assets. The resident then becomes eligible for Medicaid coverage.

Subacute Care

Serves patients needing complex care or rehabilitation. Subacute care (also known as transitional care) is defined as comprehensive inpatient care designed for someone who has an acute illness, injury or exacerbation of a disease process. It is goal oriented treatment rendered immediately after, or instead of, acute hospitalization to treat one or more specific active complex medical conditions or to administer one or more technically complex treatments, in the context of a person's underlying long-term conditions and overall situation. Subacute care may include long-term ventilator care or other procedures provided on a routine basis either at home or by trained staff at a skilled nursing facility. Subacute care is generally more intensive than traditional nursing facility care and less than acute care. It requires frequent (daily to weekly) recurrent patient assessment and review of the clinical course and treatment plan for a limited (several days to several months) time period until the condition is stabilized or a predetermined treatment course is completed.

Supplemental Security Income

Known as SSI, this program may provide monthly disability income for those who meet Social Security rules for disability who have limited income and resources. A public assistance program providing support for low-income aged, blind and disabled persons, established by Title XVI of the Social Security Act. SSI replaced state welfare programs for the aged, blind and disabled in since 1972, with a federally administered program, paying a monthly basic benefit nationwide of $284.30 for an individual and $426.40 for a couple in 1983. States may supplement this basic benefit amount.

T

Term Life Insurance

Provides coverage for individuals for a period of one or more years. Pays a death benefit only if individual dies during that term. It does not typically build cash value.

Third Party Notice

A policy provision that allows the policyholder name someone who the insurance company would notify if coverage were about to end because premiums haven't been paid. This individual can be a relative, friend, or professional such as a lawyer or accountant.

Transitional Care

Transitional care can be defined as that which is required to facilitate a shift from one disease stage and/orplace of care to another. Also known as post-acute care or subacute care, a type of short-term care provided by many long-term care facilities and hospitals which may include rehabilitation services, specialized care for certain diseases, conditions and/or post-surgical care and other services associated with the transition between the hospital and home. Residents on these units often have been hospitalized recently and typically have more complicated medical needs. The goal of subacute care is to discharge residents to their homes or to a lower level of care.

Trust

A legal title to property held by one party for the benefit of another. An arrangement in which an individual (the trustor) gives fiduciary control of property to a person or institution (the trustee) for the benefit of one or more beneficiaries. The property so held is known as a trust.

Trustor

An individual, organization or institution (such as a bank, that holds legal title to property in order to administer it for a beneficiary.

TTY

A text telephone system that allows a hearing-impaired user to type messages (data), one character at a time, to another person and read responses on a small screen. Similar to cell phone text messaging, a "read only" conversation can exist between two people who each use the equipment. An option is having a non-hearing-impaired caller utilize. This term refers to a means of sending data one character at a time. a relay service where a special operator acts as a go-between to translate the speaker's words into text and text print into voice communication.

U

Universal Life Insurance

Flexible type of policy that allows individuals to periodically adjust their premium payments and the amount of coverage.

V

Veterans

For Federal financial aid purposes such as determining dependency status, a veteran is a former member of the US Armed Forces (Army, Navy, Air Force, Marines or Coast Guard) who served on active duty and was discharged other than dishonorably (i.e., received an honorable or medical discharge).

One anonymous writer once said: "A veteran is someone who, at one point in his/her life, wrote a blank check made payable to "The United States of America," for an amount of 'up to and including my life.'"

Veterans Benefits

Depending on their service record, veterans and their dependents may be eligible for health care, military pensions, education assistance (GI Bill), housing, burial aid, life insurance, employment preferences and other benefits. Veteran applications are evaluated individually and veterans ineligible for one type of assistance may be entitled to other benefits. All former military personnel are encouraged to apply for benefits at their local VA office or by calling 800-827-1000.

Medical benefits, authorized under 38 USC 17, available to military veterans who have a Service-connected illness or injury through programs administered by the Veterans Administration (VA). Payments made by VA to veterans, or dependents of veterans.

Visiting Nurse Association

A voluntary health agency that is a not-for-profit organization providing intermittent, skilled care in the home under orders from your physician. Basic services include health supervision, education and counseling; bedside care; and carrying out of physicians' orders. Personnel include nurses and home health aides who are trained for specific tasks of personal bedside care. These agencies are committed to providing the finest home health care available, regardless of an individual's ability to pay.

W

Whole Life Insurance

Policies that build cash value and cover a person for as long as he or she lives if premiums continue to be paid.

ABOUT THE AUTHOR

Dee Marrella has experienced life as both a military and a corporate wife. As a result, she has seen much of the world and been exposed to many varied cultures. Born in Paterson, New Jersey, Dee spent twenty-plus years in the field of education in both Europe and the United States. Experiencing those different cultures afforded her the opportunity to observe first hand the vast differences in the ways caregivers interact with both young and old individuals within societies. Today she is the proud wife of retired LT. Colonel and businessman, Len Marrella, the mother of three grown daughters, and the grandmother of seven grandchildren.

Back in 1994 it was medically necessary for Dee's mother to enter a nursing home. Dee maintained a constant presence at the home. Watching so many caregivers deal with pain, love and guilt gave her the inspiration to create her first caregiving book, *Who Cares.* After two successful editions of *Who Cares*, a new book was created and entitled, *The Me You Don't Know*. This new, updated and expanded publication, *Everything About ME*, takes an entire decade of sharing and learning and provides an entirely fresh approach to future caregiving.

By preparing ahead, you create a win-win situation for all involved in your life. If you have physical or mental issues and if you find yourself, one day, in the hands of future caregivers (family, friends, strangers), **you can** have a "voice" in your future. This book allows for decision-making "**by you" not "for you.**" Your loved ones win by having peace of mind, through concrete guidance from YOU.

Everything About *ME* is a form of insurance. I call it "Love Insurance." This book insures that all individuals involved in your caregiving, one day in the future, are properly informed of what YOU want. This is an instructional manual, a guide, a diary that tells people how YOU wish to be cared for. This book is written by "the person" who knows the most about you **YOU!!** This is a celebration of who you are.

REMEMBER . . .
The opposite of love is not hate
The opposite of love is indifference.
By filling this book out, YOU prove you are not indifferent.

– Dee Marrella

PUBLISHER'S COMMENTS

All the publishers I know, hope and pray for a project to come along that really lights a fire under them and provides their audiences the most engaging experience possible. We all hope for a book that just reaches out and grabs the reader (user) and gives them the most value for the time they invest. The book that you are holding isn't fiction. It doesn't have thrilling chase scenes, nor does it have heroes that overcome evil and save the world. This book is real life and the hero is YOU.

In the society we live in, it is becoming rare to find close-knit families, adult children who live geographically close to their parents and siblings, or a real feeling of community. As we age, such things become more important. And when we think about our own future such as the possibility of being cared for by others, we tend to imagine that we'll be cared for by members of our immediate family (such as a surviving spouse or adult children). This may becoming more of a dream than a reality. Statistics strongly indicate that the majority of us will be cared for by strangers people outside our family people who do not know who we are.

We have found that caring for others is a valuable gift that we an give one that gives meaning to family and friends during the last years (of days) of their lives. We have also found that caring for others gives us a better feeling about ourselves. There really is meaning to giving of oneself and ones' time. However, while we are caring for others, the vast majority of us fail to "think" or "consider that one day, we'll be in need of care. And when that day comes, will we be prepared?

The answer isn't good: "NO." Most Americans do not think about how they will be cared for in the future. Sure, we purchase life insurance. We buy car, home, property, and health insurance. We even insure cell phones and flat screen TV's against damage. We buy into retirement plans and feed investments. We purchase retirement homes. BUT…do we really give consideration to who will be caring for our medical needs, feeding us, cleaning us, spending time reading with us? Most of us don't.

Dee Marrella has created the most engaging means for YOU to "tell" those people in your future "everything about yourself." From birth through school, from the type of jobs you've held to the hobbies you spend your private time working on, Everything About ME provides you an opportunity to write down the key facts the most important bits of data about YOU. Since few of us actually talk with our spouses about such topics (let alone our children), there are few people (if any) who really know anything, in depth, about ourselves.

Consider that one day you might wake up, let's say, from a coma. You don't know your surroundings. The smells are different than you're used to. The TV in the room is on, but it is showing a Clint Eastwood movie and doesn't anyone know that you just hate Clint Eastwood movies? Someone walks by and smiles at you. You don't recognize their face. And, they don't speak to you. They just walk by. As you follow them, you decide to say something ask a question. BUT, to your surprise, you can't speak. You've had a stroke and can't move a part of your body, and your voice is silent.

This is just one example of when "the book" (Everything About ME) comes into play.

If you had completed the pages of this book. If you had discussed your thoughts and comments with your spouse, adult children, other family, and friends (including an attorney and your physician), there would be a number of people who had become educated about who you are and who you were (in your younger days).

Dee Marrella has set up a process whereby YOU can answer questions, tell people about your "likes" and "dislikes," let the world in on who you were back in elementary school, the first musical instrument you attempted to play, the kinds of movies you enjoy, foods that really are your favorites and those you just hate. Without this information readily available in one location, in one format, there is little possibility that anyone will completely know who you are. AND, if you can't speak and tell them, how will they find out?

Rather than becoming a name, an account number, a person with ten medications to take each day, and little else, wouldn't you prefer that those who care for you in the future know who you are? Wouldn't you want to have a voice in your future care? Wouldn't you want people to know how you feel about important issues, such as: life support, organ transplants, healthcare professionals that you prefer take care of you, and how you'd like your funeral to be handled?

All of this can now be under your control. YOU have a copy of one of the most important books published. And when you've completed filling out the pages, you will have a gift for your future caregivers that no one else could have produced. You are the only one. You have the answers. Aren't you glad that you've taken the time to share yourself with the future? Those who care for you will be very pleased.

Your journey is about t begin. Enjoy the trip. And…one day, appreciate the results. YOU are doing a great thing for yourself.

Dennis McClellan, Publisher
DC Press

*If you found this book thought provoking and would like to
have Dee Marrella speak to your organization,
please feel free to contact her at:*

Dee Marrella

Phone: 610.478.3000
Fax: 610.478.3001
dee@deemarrella.com
www.deemarrella.com

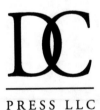

PRESS LLC

www. focusonethics.com
www.dcpressbooks.com

PHOTOGRAPH OF ME

As I would like to be remembered

Name: _____

PLACE
PHOTO
HERE